95

/00

THE PATIENT'S GUIDE TO
HOMEOPATHIC
MEDICINE

THE PATIENT'S GUIDE TO HOMEOPATHIC MEDICINE

ROBERT ULLMAN, N.D.

JUDYTH REICHENBERG-ULLMAN, N.D., M.S.W.

PICNIC POINT PRESS

EDMONDS, WASHINGTON

Publisher's Cataloging in Publication

Ullman, Robert W., 1951 –
        The patient's guide to homeopathic medicine / Robert Ullman and Judyth Reichenberg–Ullman.
        p. cm.
        Includes bibliographical references and index.
        ISBN 0-9640654-2-8

        1. Homeopathy.   I. Reichenberg–Ullman, Judyth. II. Title.
    RX71.U55 1995   615.5'32'03
                                           QB195-20062

Designed by Kate L. Thompson.

This book is intended for educational purposes only. It is not intended for purposes of self-diagnosis or self-treatment. Further, it is not intended to diagnose, treat, give medical advice for a specific condition, or in any way to replace the services of a qualified medical professional.

ISBN 0-9640654-2-8

LCCN 94-90871

99 98 97 5 4

**Picnic Point Press
131 Third Ave. N., Suite B
Edmonds, WA 98020
(206) 233-1155**

ACKNOWLEDGMENTS

SPECIAL THANKS to Miranda Castro, for her helpful suggestions and publishing savvy, and for connecting us with her excellent editor, Hazel Orme, to whom we are very grateful. We thank Marilyn Osterman, our copy editor, for her careful attention to detail and Kate Thompson, our book designer, for her excellent work on our cover, book interior, and logo. We particularly thank Roger Morrison for writing the foreword and for sharing his self-publishing experience and thank his lovely wife and colleague Nancy Herrick for her kind encouragement. We also thank Barry and Joyce Vissell for sharing their love and support for our relationship and our book.

Many thanks to all of you who reviewed our manuscript and gave us helpful feedback including Dr. Rajan Sankaran, George Vithoulkas, Dr. Jennifer Jacobs, John Clancey, Jay Borneman, Dr. William Shevin, Dr. Karen Fuller, Linda DeBoer, Steve and Randa Cleaves, Dr. Michael Traub, Julian Winston, Dr. Amy Haines, Dr. Ellen Goldman, Stacy Hartog, Dana Ullman, Dr. Stephen Messer, Dr. Stephen King, Dr. Sheryl Kipnis, Peggy Chipkin, and Mort Yanow.

To all of you we forgot to mention, our sincerest gratitude for your support.

DEDICATION

We dedicate this book to all those who made it possible: To Samuel Hahnemann for his brilliance, courage, and inspiration; To all of our teachers of homeopathy for their wisdom; To homeopaths everywhere for their dedication and compassion; To our colleagues and friends, who have supported this project from beginning to end; To our patients, who continue to be our greatest teachers of homeopathy; To our parents for their love, prayers, and confidence in all of our endeavors.

TABLE OF CONTENTS

FOREWORD

BY ROGER MORRISON, M.D.

IT IS A GREAT PLEASURE to introduce this wonderful book to the public and to my professional colleagues. The homeopathic community has needed such a book for many years. This is because *The Patient's Guide to Homeopathic Medicine* is the first book tailored exactly to the needs of homeopaths and their patients. While there exist many fine introductory books on homeopathy, most offer explanations of homeopathy without the details of how it works from inside the healing process. This is akin to selling a computer without a manual. Now, for the first time, homeopathic patients have a user's manual.

The purpose of this book is to make the homeopathic process understandable to the patient. The chapters on the homeopathic interview and dos and don'ts for patients are unique in homeopathic books addressed to the general public. These chapters give truly in-depth explanations to the questions patients commonly ask in homeopathic practice. As knowledge empowers, this book will empower our patients, making them partners in treatment rather than passive participants.

Of almost equal importance with the explanatory portion of this book is its friendly and supportive tone. The book invites the patient into the perspective of the trained homeopath or the seasoned homeopathic patient. The authors evoke the passion and wonder every experienced physician feels for this magnificent healing art. This book gives the patient an idea of the commitment and love that each homeopath has for his art. The authors communicate the full capacity for healing in our lives and help the patient understand the full scope of the truly miraculous changes that homeopathy offers.

Judyth and Robert are known throughout the homeopathic community for their commitment to excellence, their compassion toward their patients, and their dedication to homeopathic education. The authors are regular contributors to *Resonance,* the magazine of the International Foundation for Homeopathy; the *Townsend Letter for Doctors*; and also write for *Simillimum,* the journal of the Homeopathic Association of Naturopathic Physicians. Both authors are licensed naturopathic physicians have been teachers of repute in naturopathic medical schools, and are instructors in the International Foundation for Homeopathy's professional course. It is a rare event when two such proficient and recognized physicians take time to look through their patient's eyes and carefully outline homeopathy from this perspective.

Homeopathy is one of the most dynamic forms of medicine in the world today, capable of producing profound, lasting healing.

INTRODUCTION

HOMEOPATHY IS ONE of the most dynamic forms of medicine in the world today, capable of producing profound, lasting healing. It is enjoying growing recognition worldwide, and the media is devoting more coverage to homeopathy than ever before. The National Institutes of Health recently included homeopathy as an area of alternative medicine that merits further research. We feel fortunate to be part of a new generation of homeopaths who are committed to promoting and perpetuating this highly effective form of natural medicine.

Over the past ten years, we have treated thousands of patients in our homeopathic practices. In this book, we answer the questions that patients commonly ask about homeopathy. The result is a concise and practical guide to homeopathic treatment.

Informed patients are more likely to follow through with homeopathic treatment and derive benefit from it. They can better understand and follow their practitioners' instructions. They pay closer attention to their symptoms and communicate them more clearly to their homeopaths. They are also more knowledgeable about avoiding anything that might interfere with their treatment.

If patients derive more benefit from their homeopathic treatment because of the information they receive here, this book will have achieved its purpose. We hope that, through homeopathy, as well as through other forms of healing, human suffering can be greatly alleviated. As satisfied patients share their enthusiasm with their family and friends, more and more people can be helped by homeopathy.

The identities of patients referred to in this book have been disguised to protect their privacy. We alternate "he" and "she" for the purpose of equality of gender reference.

More books and articles have been published about homeopathy in the last five years than in the preceding fifty.

HOMEOPATHY:
ROOTS AND RENAISSANCE

FOR OVER TWO HUNDRED YEARS, people all over the world have found the solutions to their health problems through homeopathy. If you are new to homeopathy, you may be asking yourself, "What *is* homeopathy?" "Where did it come from?" Let's start at the beginning.

Samuel Hahnemann, The Founder of Homeopathy

Samuel Hahnemann (1755-1843) was a German scholar, physician, and chemist. He was fluent in at least seven languages and well versed in the medical thought of his day. Hahnemann was appalled by the often dangerous and ineffective methods of healing used by his contemporaries. Treatments such as vomiting, purging, sweating, bloodletting, applying leeches, and using poisonous substances, like mercury and arsenic, in large doses often prolonged the patients' suffering before finally killing them. George Washington was treated with repeated bloodletting in an attempt to cure a fever. The "cure" killed him.

Prior to his discovery of homeopathy, Hahnemann gave up the practice of medicine because he could no longer bear to injure his patients or prolong their illnesses. He chose instead to make his living as a medical translator.

Hahnemann Discovers Homeopathy

Hahnemann was a tireless student of the medical literature and a relentless investigator. While translating a book on medicinal substances by William Cullen, an eminent Scottish physician, Hahnemann questioned why *Cinchona* bark (from which quinine was later derived) could cure malaria. Cullen's explanation that the bark cured malaria because of its bitter taste did not satisfy Hahnemann. He reasoned that if *Cinchona* bark's curative properties were based solely on its bitterness, then other bitter substances should be equally curative, which he knew from his clinical experience was not the case. He decided to take an extract of the bark himself to experience its effects firsthand. Hahnemann found that upon taking successive doses of the medicine, he developed chills, weakness, and sweats. These, he realized, were very similar to the actual symptoms of malaria.

From this experiment, Hahnemann recognized the principle that like cures like. This principle, called *the law of similars,* is not new. Ancient healers such as Charaka in India (c.1000 B.C.), Hippocrates in Greece (c.400 B.C.), and Paracelsus, the medieval European physician, referred to this principle in their writings. Hahnemann theorized that if *Cinchona* bark could produce symptoms similar to malaria and could also cure malaria, then the same could be true of other substances as well. Hahnemann expanded this ancient idea into a complete medical system for the first time. He coined the term *homeopathy,* from the Greek roots for similar and suffering to describe the new system that he evolved from the law of similars.

He began to test many other natural or medicinal substances such as *Belladonna, Arsenic, Mercury*, and *Sulphur* to see the range of symptoms that each substance could produce in a healthy person. These experiments, conducted on himself, family, friends, and students, were known as *provings.* Hahnemann gradually built up a working knowledge of a number of medicines, called *materia medica*, which he found to be highly effective with patients.

Hahnemann began to write about his homeopathic experiments as early as 1792, but his major work on homeopathic philosophy and treatment, the *Organon of Medicine*, was not published until 1810. Five editions of the *Organon* were published between 1810 and 1843 as Hahnemann kept experimenting and improving the medical art that he had developed. A sixth edition was published in 1921, more than 75 years after his death.

The physicians of Hahnemann's time strongly opposed his new system of medicine, in part because it was a radical change from the orthodoxy of the time, but also because its success provided significant competition. Hahnemann was forced to leave the city of Leipzig, the bastion of German medical learning, because his ideas were too unconventional for most of his colleagues.

Over the course of his life, Hahnemann treated thousands of patients, including many highly respected intellectuals, artists, and government officials in Germany and France. He personally proved almost a hundred medicines before his death at the age of 88. By that time, he had finally received the recognition he deserved for his groundbreaking discoveries.

The Rise and Decline of Homeopathy

Even before Hahnemann's death, homeopathy had spread from Germany and France throughout Europe and to the United States. The first homeopathic medical school was established in the United States in 1836 in Allentown, Pennsylvania. The American Institute of Homeopathy, the first national homeopathic organization, was founded in 1844. Homeopathy achieved great recognition for its success in treating epidemics such as cholera, scarlet fever, and yellow fever. By the turn of the century, approximately one in five physicians was a homeopath. More than one hundred homeopathic hospitals, over twenty homeopathic medical schools, and at least a thousand homeopathic pharmacies flourished in the United States at that time. [1]

Despite its clinical success, there was considerable opposition to homeopathy, both in Europe and the United States. The American Medical Association was founded in 1846, in opposition to the homeopaths. State medical societies in the United States prohibited their members from referring to, or even consulting with, a homeopath. The pharmaceutical companies, standing to lose considerable profits if inexpensive homeopathic medicines became too popular, published articles disparaging the new medical system. Many orthodox physicians felt threatened by the growing acceptance of homeopathy.

In 1910, the Carnegie Foundation hired Abraham Flexner to evaluate all of the medical schools in the United States to determine which would receive funding from the foundation. Flexner gave the homeopathic medical schools poor ratings, largely because they did not emphasize laboratory facilities. Homeopathic schools lost foundation support and state licensing boards began to use the Flexner report to determine which graduates could take licensing exams. As a result, homeopathy nearly died in the United States by the mid-twentieth century.

Gradually all of the homeopathic medical schools were forced out of business or converted to conventional medical institutions. With the advent of modern medicines such as sulfa drugs and penicillin, the "wonder drugs" of the 1940's, public interest turned to the new pharmaceutical drugs and support of homeopathy waned dramatically. By 1950, there were no homeopathic medical schools left in the United States and there were only a few dedicated practitioners remaining. The opportunity to learn homeopathy in the United States was nearly lost. During the 1960's a relatively small, but dedicated, group of practitioners and patients continued to use homeopathy. One of the main ways that the homeopathic tradition was preserved was through study groups, in which lay people studied homeopathy together on a regular basis. Today these study groups are more widespread than ever and many are coordinated by the National Center for Homeopathy. (See the Appendix for more information.)

Homeopathic Renaissance and Research

During the late 1960's, interest in alternative lifestyles and medicine began to blossom. Many people were searching for a more natural, healthy way to live. Vitamins, herbs, homeopathy, and other forms of natural healing began to be in demand and by the late 1970's homeopathy began to experience a resurgence in the United States.

Once again, seminars and training programs were offered to serious students of homeopathy. George Vithoulkas, an innovative Greek homeopath, was a primary influence in training a new generation of homeopaths. Vithoulkas had acquired vast experience from having treated thousands of patients from all over Europe at his homeopathic clinic in Athens. He synthesized his tremendous clinical knowledge into a practical textbook, *The Science of Homeopathy*. Enthusiastic North American homeopaths developed clinics and homeopathic treatment began to be available in a few areas of the United States and Canada. It is some of these same homeopaths, who have now practiced homeopathy for ten to twenty years, who provide much of the homeopathic education in this country today.

More books and articles have been published about homeopathy in the last five years than in the preceding fifty. There are more than one thousand medically-trained homeopaths now practicing in the United States, including medical doctors, osteopathic physicians, naturopathic physicians, chiropractors, physician assistants, acupuncturists, dentists, nurses, nurse practitioners, and veterinarians. In addition, a growing number of unlicensed, yet well-trained homeopathic practititioners, are currently seeking certification.

In 1992, the National Institutes of Health appointed a group of respected health professionals to evaluate the effectiveness of alternative therapies, including homeopathy. This was a breakthrough towards mainstream acceptance of homeopathy and other effective alternative therapies. A survey in the January 28, 1993, issue of the *New England Journal of Medicine* revealed that more than one-third of Americans were using some form of alternative medicine, including homeopathy. The total number of visits to alternative practitioners was greater than those to primary care physicians.[2]

Landmark research studies in the efficacy of homeopathic medicine were published in two highly prestigious medical journals in 1994. Jennifer Jacobs, M.D., M.P.H. conducted a randomized clinical trial of children with acute childhood diarrhea in Nicaragua. The study, published in *Pediatrics*, indicated a statistically significant decrease in duration of the diarrhea and encouraged further homeopathic research.[3] David Reilly, M.D., of Glasgow, Scotland, undertook a clinical study of patients with allergic asthma. This study, published in *The Lancet*, also demonstrated the efficacy of homeopathy.[4] These studies are hopefully the first of many to be published in conventional medical journals and to confirm the clinical effectiveness of homeopathy.

Homeopathic Training

Although there are still no accredited homeopathic colleges in the United States, there are a growing number of opportunities for homeopathic education. Homeopathy is an integral part of the curriculum at all three colleges of naturopathic medicine: Bastyr University, the National College of Naturopathic Medicine, and the

Southwest College of Naturopathic Medicine. These three colleges are the only medical degree programs that include a significant amount of homeopathy in their training. The Hahnemann College of Homeopathy, the International Foundation for Homeopathy, the National Center for Homeopathy, and the New England School of Homeopathy offer postgraduate programs for licensed health care professionals.

The International Foundation for Homeopathy, the Homeopathic Academy of Naturopathic Physicians, the National Center for Homeopathy, and the American Institute of Homeopathy are all very active in supporting the spread of homeopathy in the United States. Each of these organizations publishes a homeopathic journal and sponsors an annual conference. The National Center for Homeopathy, the Atlantic Academy of Homeopathy, the Pacific Academy of Homeopathy, and the New England School of Homeopathy all offer courses for nonprofessionals.

Homeopathy Throughout The World

Homeopathy is widely practiced in India, England, France, Germany, Mexico, and South America, and is gaining acceptance among conventional medical practitioners in Western Europe. In England, homeopathy has been used by the royal family since 1830. There are more than twenty homeopathic schools or part-time courses there including a course for medical doctors at the Royal London Homeopathic Hospital. In England, there are many registered professional homeopaths who are members of the Society of Homeopaths. A recent study on the attitudes of British physicians to complementary medicine found that 42 percent refer to homeopaths.[5] In France, over 11,000 physicians use homeopathic medicines, which are dispensed by more than 20,000 pharmacies. Twenty-five percent of the French people have been treated homeopathically.[6] Postgraduate homeopathic courses are offered throughout Europe, particularly in Belgium, Germany, France and Greece. Standards for education in homeopathy and a model course curriculum are being formulated and promoted by the European and International Councils for Classical Homeopathy. In India, as part of the legacy of British colonialism, there are 120 homeopathic medical colleges and as many as 100,000 homeopathic practitioners. The Indian government sponsors nineteen medical colleges and a number of homeopathic hospitals.[7]

Notes

1 Ullman, Dana, *Discovering Homeopathy-Medicine for the 21st Century.* Berkeley: North Atlantic Books, 1988, pg. 40.

2 Eisenberg DM, Kessler RC, Foster C, Norlock FE, Calkins, DR, and Delbanco, TL., "Unconventional Medicine in the United States." *N Engl J Med* 1993; 328:246-252.

3 Jacobs J, Jimennez M, Gloyd S, Gale J, and Crothers D., "Treatment of Acute Childhood Diarrhea With Homeopathic Medicine: A Randomized Clinical Trial in Nicatagua." *Ped* 1994; 93:719-725.

4 Reilly D, Taylor MA, Beattie NG, Campbell JH, McSharry C, Aitchison TC, Carter R, and Stevenson RD., "Is Evidence for Homeopathy Reproducible?" *Lancet* 1994; 344: 1601-1606.

5 Wharton R, Lewith G., "Complementary Medicine and the General Practitioner." *Brit Med J* 1986; 292:1498-1500.

6 Ullman, op cit., pg. 48.

7 Ibid.

*Homeopaths treat people,
not diagnoses.*

WHAT IN THE WORLD
IS HOMEOPATHY?

The Law of Similars

Homeopathy uses natural substances that can *cause* symptoms in a healthy person to *cure* similar symptoms in a person who is ill. Can you remember the last time you were stung by a bee? The stinging, burning pain, swelling, heat, and redness are probably etched in your memory. These are the symptoms that you experience when an angry bee injects its venom into your healthy body. How can a poisonous substance like bee venom *(Apis mellifica)* be used as a medicine? It is precisely the fact that it *causes* symptoms that makes it useful as a medicine. Bee venom, when used as a homeopathic medicine, can relieve the pain and discomfort of bee stings as well as other illnesses that have similar symptoms. People suffering from conjunctivitis (pink eye), who complain of stinging or burning pain, redness and swelling of the eyelids, often benefit from *Apis*. The type of arthritis that is hot, red, and swollen with stinging pains may also be cured or helped by a dose of homeopathic bee venom.

If you think about the law of similars, you may realize how different it is from the philosophy of conventional medicine. Most of us in Western society have been taught to believe that the only way to eliminate a bacterial infection is with antibiotics. "Anti" means against. The use of antibiotics is based on the belief that there is a battle being waged in the body which must be won, and that the body is unable to win it without the antibiotics. Antibiotics tend to kill microorganisms that are associated with disease or interfere with their reproduction. This may allow the body to recover from the illness.

A homeopath might also say that the body needs help in fighting the infection, but homeopathy gives that assistance in a different way. When a homeopathic remedy is given, the symptom pattern of the remedy matches the symptoms of the disease and strengthens the body's own ability to fight the infection and restore balance. Homeopathic theory says that the real cause of an infection is not the microorganism, but the set of conditions in a person's body that provides an environment in which the viruses or bacteria can survive and multiply. If you can restore the natural ecology of the body with homeopathy, the microorganisms will no longer be able to create disease.

In the conventional medical approach, if the stomach is producing too much hydrochloric acid, a drug is given which reduces the stomach's ability to secrete acid. A person suffering from allergies is given an antihistamine, which prevents the release of histamine, the chemical secreted by the mucous membranes in response to an allergen. Steroids, such as hydrocortisone, are used to suppress inflammatory responses.

It may sound like a good idea to fight *against* invading organisms or processes that cause damage to the body. Antibiotics, anti-inflammatories, antacids, antifungals, and antihistamines do produce effects and on the surface relieve illness. Over time, however, these medications may produce mild to severe side effects. The result may be only temporary or superficial healing. These drugs may ultimately cause more serious problems than they cure. Homeopathy, on the other hand, works *with* the body rather than *against* it.

Illness, Balance and Health

To a homeopath, illness is an energy imbalance that occurs first at the most fundamental levels of the person. This underlying imbalance is the cause of disease and shows itself eventually in the body as symptoms, which are created by the body in the process of trying to correct the imbalance. It is the imbalance itself that homeopathy addresses, using the symptoms as a guide to the natural substance that can be of assistance in the process.

If you are in perfect balance, which is unusual, you will not develop any symptoms. If you are totally healthy, you are free of pain and physical symptoms, have plenty of energy, think clearly, experience happiness and a passion for life, and genuinely care about others. You are free to be yourself and to express your creativity.

Homeopathy attempts to bring each individual to the highest level of health possible on the physical, mental, and emotional levels. Samuel Hahnemann affirmed, "The highest ideal of cure is to restore health rapidly, gently, permanently... in the shortest, surest, least harmful way according to clearly comprehensible principles..." [1]

You may have felt healthier, happier, and more energetic at some earlier time in your life. You may believe that you're just getting old and that good health is no longer possible for you. Homeopathy can often restore your health and vitality beyond your expectations.

The Vital Force and the Defense Mechanism

The dynamic balance of all the functions of your body within the narrow range that maintains life and health is known as homeostasis. Homeostasis means keeping things static or constant. Imagine that your body is a gyroscope. As long as the gyroscope is spinning vigorously, it will stay in balance, even though outside forces may try to topple it. If you push it to one side, it will return to its upright position naturally.

Homeostatic and self-regulatory mechanisms constantly maintain the physiology of the body. Numerous feedback loops in the body stimulate necessary adjustments in your physiology. When the carbon dioxide content of your blood begins to rise, you breathe more deeply or you begin to yawn. When you drink too much coffee or beer, urination is increased to decrease the liquid volume in your body. When your immune system recognizes a protein that is foreign to your system, antibodies are produced to take the protein out of circulation before it can do any damage.

These self-regulatory mechanisms operate in an organized fashion, but the organizing principle that causes them to function is difficult to observe directly. Physiologists assume that there is an underlying principle because the body continues to live, think, eat, digest, reproduce, and move. When the body fails to do these things, we consider a person to be dead. So what is the difference between being alive and being dead?

Homeopaths believe that, as long as you are alive, there exists within you a living, intelligent energy that is responsible for healing and maintaining balance in your body, mind, and emotions. This energy is called the *vital force*. The idea has been shared by many cultures throughout the world, using names such as *ki, prana, mana,* and *life force.* Although the vital force is intangible, its effects are readily apparent.

The *defense mechanism* is the aspect of the vital force that is responsible for preventing illness and bringing all of your systems back into equilibrium. It helps your body repel invading organisms and keeps all of your internal biological functions running smoothly.

The *immune system* is the physical aspect of the defense mechanism. It uses specialized cells and tissues to neutralize, destroy, or immobilize any foreign cells or tissues.

The defense mechanism is not just physical; there are also mental and emotional aspects of the defense mechanism. It is just as responsible for healing the grief from a death in the family, or the confusion and delusions of the schizophrenic mind, as it is for healing a bruised toe, a cold, or an ulcer. It helps you to release anger, grief, and sadness; to forgive those who have hurt you; and to restore your emotional balance. It can also help you regain mental concentration, clarity of thought, and good memory.

You can help strengthen your defense mechanism and prevent minor health problems from becoming more serious if you pay attention to the messages your body is communicating to you. When your defense mechanism cannot prevent a situation, you begin to notice warning signals. You may get a slight sore throat, then a runny nose, then aches and pains, and then a fever. These are signs from the defense mechanism prompting you to pay attention and restore your health. It is your responsibility to take over. You can get more rest, eat lightly, take Vitamin C, and reduce the stress in your life. Suppose that in the process of defending you, however, the body keeps generating more symptoms that become increasingly severe, and do not go away. This is when homeopathy can help.

The Importance of Symptoms

Common symptoms such as pain, inflammation, fever, swelling, and changes in perspiration, urination, sleep, hunger, and thirst, often point to an imbalance in the body. Without symptoms, you would never know that you were ill and your homeopath could not assist you in getting better.

Your homeopath takes a careful case history and performs a physical examination when necessary. She observes you, listens to all of your symptoms, then uses them to select a homeopathic remedy. The more peculiar and unusual your symptoms are, the easier it is to find a medicine that uniquely matches them.

Local illnesses without symptoms, such as a brain tumor, rectal polyps, breast lumps, or cancer of the cervix often go undetected for a long time, unless discovered on routine physical examination. Your defense mechanism may not yet have found a way to bring the problem to your attention or to correct it. Sometimes the body generates other symptoms, along with the hidden illness, which you *can* notice. These symptoms often lead your homeopath to discover the illness and to prescribe a remedy which will cure it.

Joan

32, complained of a skin rash on her face. As part of her routine physical exam, a Pap smear, which was several years overdue, was recommended. The Pap smear results indicated significant precancerous cell changes in her cervix (cervical dysplasia). Although the cervical dysplasia was asymptomatic, the rash led her to seek treatment. Through homeopathy and other natural therapies, both the rash and the cervical dysplasia were cured.

The Simillimum

Homeopaths prescribe only one remedy at a time. This remedy, which best matches your symptoms, is called the *simillimum*. There may be other homeopathic remedies that will have an effect on your symptoms, but there is no other remedy that will work as well. The simillimum is the remedy that will cure your symptoms, based on the principle of like cures like.

At another time, your body might produce a different set of symptoms and require another remedy. This new remedy would be the simillimum *at that time*. In some cases, one remedy is all a person ever needs to remain healthy. Generally, during treatment for chronic illness, which is called *constitutional treatment*, more than one remedy may be needed over time to help you stay healthy. If the pattern of your symptoms changes enough to fall outside the scope of the original remedy, a new remedy is needed.

Individualization of Treatment

Homeopaths treat people, not diagnoses. When you are ill, your illness has its own unique pattern of symptoms. You will tend to get those illnesses that result from the particular pattern of imbalance that is unique to your personal heredity and environmental influences. If you have a weakness in the urinary system, you may develop symptoms of bladder infections or kidney disease. If your skin is the problem, you may be prone to rashes, herpes or warts. If the digestive system is the focus, you may suffer from ulcers, constipation or hemorrhoids. Patterns of certain illnesses may run in your family and be passed on from generation to generation.

People with the same diagnosis will *not* all need the same homeopathic remedy. There is no one homeopathic treatment, for instance, for flu. Your homeopath needs to know *whose* flu is being treated. *Your* flu requires a homeopathic medicine that matches *your* particular pattern of symptoms. Someone else's flu will respond to an entirely different homeopathic remedy.

You may have a flu that comes on right after exposure to a cold, dry wind. Suddenly, you develop a high fever. You notice, to your surprise, that one cheek is pale and the other red. You sneeze violently, your nose runs like a faucet, and you have a nagging, dry, croupy cough. You feel uncharacteristically restless. You have a strong fear that you might get worse, even die, because your symptoms have come on so suddenly and violently. Your mouth is bone dry and you can't drink enough water. You feel chilled to the core. You need the homeopathic remedy *Aconitum napellus,* which will rapidly restore your health.

Suppose your neighbor gets a flu which comes on gradually, over a few days. Just before she became sick, she was very nervous about giving a speech in front of five hundred people. She feels great exhaustion and can hardly keep her eyes open, or even move. She experiences icy chills up and down her spine. Her mouth feels like cotton, but she's not thirsty. Her body aches all over, like she's been carrying a fifty pound backpack. Her arms and legs feel terribly heavy. Her limbs tremble. She feels dizzy, drowsy, droopy and dull. Although your neighbor's diagnosis would also be influenza, she needs a different homeopathic medicine. *Gelsemium sempervirens* will not only cure her flu, but may help her stage fright as well.

The following three cases of patients with hay fever show how each individual set of symptoms, even with the same diagnosis, can lead a homeopath to prescribe very different homeopathic medicines.

Prabha

Prabha was a 30 year old East Indian woman who was led to homeopathy because of hay fever. Her bouts normally lasted all spring until mid or late summer. She awoke in the morning with a dry cough, congestion in the upper lungs, and slight wheezing. During the day she complained of terrible itching in the ears, Eustachian tubes, and some itching in the throat, nose, and eyes. She had occasional sneezing, runny nose, and dry eyes. The symptoms lasted throughout the day and were better when she was indoors. We gave Prabha *Nux vomica* because of the dry cough with wheezing on waking, combined with the sneezing and itching inside the nose. She received the remedy in the spring, with great benefit. She continued to take it occasionally, as needed, during the summer. When she returned to us the following spring, with the same symptoms, she was again given *Nux vomica*.

Erik

Erik, a young Norwegian man, had been bothered by hay fever since the age of five. It was usually worse in the summer, but a severe attack in late March prompted him to see a homeopath for the first time. His main problem was frequent, violent, fitful sneezing, which occurred every so often. He had a watery, runny nose, causing him to "run around with a handkerchief all the time." The skin under his nose became red and sore. His eyes were itchy, dry, and irritated. His nose was stuffy, whether he was indoors or out. His forehead itched. Erik found himself lethargic with the hay fever and he had slept ten hours the night before. This was extremely unusual for him since he was generally a very high energy person. Since the hay fever began, he was irritable and felt victimized by this acute illness. Erik was given *Sabadilla*, a remedy made from a Mexican grass, which is helpful for spasmodic sneezing, nasal congestion, itching inside the nose, and profuse watery nasal discharge. The sneezing and itching were relieved completely within two days. He briefly experienced a swelling of the nasal passages, which passed.

Todd

Todd, a 26 year old computer programmer, lamented, "I'm allergic to everything that's not food during hay fever season!" His nose ran all the time. He was using half a box of tissue a day. His eyes were itchy, puffy, and watery. He suffered from a post-nasal drip which made his throat sore. His sinuses sometimes swelled with the hay fever, causing a pressing headache. His symptoms were definitely worse outdoors. He was generally tired and wiped out with the hay fever. In the past it had lasted on and off for four months. This time he saw his homeopath after only a few days since this was his worst bout ever. He reported that he had "tried everything" orthodox medicine had to offer him. Todd received *Allium cepa* (onion). (Think about what happens to you when you slice an onion, and you'll know just the kind of hay fever which needs *Allium cepa*. It works for a hay fever, or a cold, that runs like a faucet, with itchy, watery eyes and lots of sneezing.) Todd called three days later to say his nose was no longer running. The first day after starting the remedy, he experienced lots of sneezing, which passed quickly. Then he had a few mild headaches and pressure behind his eyes. By the time he called, all of the symptoms had gone away.

Treating the Underlying Cause of Illness

Homeopaths find that the root of illness, even if the symptoms are only physical, often begins from a mental or emotional trauma. The homeopath searches for the *state* of each individual that allows that person to be susceptible to particular symptoms. This state gives rise to a vulnerability that can subsequently result in disease. The state occurs on a mental/emotional level, however the repercussions can occur on any level.

Each homeopathic medicine is characterized by a particular state of mind. Each person, at any given point in time, also experiences a particular state. This state reflects that individual's response to the world around him and permeates how that person acts, talks, thinks, and feels. Imagine that a young boy goes on a rafting trip with his father and older brother. The rapids become very swift, the raft overturns, and his brother is thrown off the raft into the swirling water. The older brother screams at him to reach out to him, but he is frozen in terror. The brother is carried by the current and drowns. The young man feels an overpowering sense of helplessness and guilt. His recurrent thoughts about his brother become an obsession. He replays the event over and over in his mind, wondering if he could have saved his brother. He dreams again and again of the drowning scene. His parents and friends reassure him that he did all he could, but he doesn't believe them. He begins to feel that he is being punished by God for having failed to save his brother. This belief that he deserves punishment extends to each area of his life. His relationships and business ventures fail. Nothing brings him happiness. He may even carry this belief to his grave. This particular state is represented by the homeopathic medicine *Kali bromatum* (potassium bromate). It can alleviate this deep-seated belief that one deserves divine wrath. If this medicine were given to this man, his desperate state could be alleviated and he would come to understand and believe that he had done all he could to help his brother.

In the same way, there is a homeopathic medicine for every state that a person might experience. Each of us experiences some state which is limiting to us in some way. These states, if untreated, are often passed on from one generation to another. The homeopathic medicine, *Aurum metallicum* (gold) can be helpful for people who are deeply depressed with self-destructive tendencies, such as chronic alcoholics. Such a state may predispose not only to profound depressive states, but also to a number of physical complaints such as sinus problems, bone pain, and sensitivity to light. By understanding the state of the person, homeopaths are able to treat body, mind, and emotions simultaneously.

Casey

A mother brought in her 10 year old son Casey for help with his excessive worrying, particularly about the family finances. He was also afraid that something bad would happen to his mother and she might die. This fear had begun right after he got his neck caught in the window of the car for a minute as his mother was rolling it up. It was the panic which Casey experienced so briefly that triggered a prolonged state of fear and anxiety. This child was given homeopathic *Aconitum napellus,* and his fear was relieved.

Dynamic Healing Through Homeopathy

The simillimum catalyzes a dynamic process of healing. In acute illnesses, your symptoms may disappear within minutes or hours. For example, a boy awakens screaming in pain in the middle of the night with a fever of 103 degrees, complaining of terrible pain in his right ear. The parents desperately want to relieve their son's discomfort. If the rest of his symptoms fit the homeopathic remedy, *Belladonna* (deadly nightshade), he will usually fall right asleep and wake up the next morning as if nothing had happened. The parents are often surprised at how rapidly the healing occurs.

In chronic illnesses, the recovery may take longer. A patient with longstanding migraines may find that her headaches become less frequent and milder within a week or two of beginning homeopathic treatment, but they may not go away completely for one or more months. Patients suffering from severe arthritis or multiple sclerosis may find some relief very quickly, but the healing will continue to occur over months or years until their symptoms and overall well-being are stabilized and significantly improved.

Homeopathy can also produce dynamic changes on the mental and emotional levels. A woman who has held in her anger and humiliation from being a victim of incest as a child may find, with homeopathic treatment, that she is finally able to express her rage in a healthy way. A man who has experienced panic attacks so severe that he cannot shop in the supermarket, can, with homeopathy, often regain his peace of mind and once again lead a normal life. Even deep mental and emotional imbalances such as depression, attention deficit disorder, extreme jealousy, and compulsive handwashing, frequently respond very well to homeopathy.

If the simillimum is found, cure will result even if your symptoms have persisted for a number of years. Homeopathy taps the inherent power of the vital force within each person to bring about healing and lasting change. Discovering the correct remedy is like finding just the right key for a lock. Even if the door has been closed for years, once the key is found, it opens. Patients and homeopaths alike are continually amazed at the power of homeopathic medicines.

Suppression Versus Cure

Suppression occurs when a treatment apparently removes symptoms on one level, but causes them to appear at a different, often deeper, level. If the body is prevented from expressing symptoms on a more superficial level, it may have no other recourse than to generate symptoms at a deeper one. Many common treatments in orthodox medicine, such as hydrocortisone cream for eczema, laser treatment for venereal warts, or antihistamines for allergy-induced nasal discharge, are potentially suppressive. Some people can receive these conventional medications and interventions without experiencing suppression. For others, the treatment will make the person even sicker.

Helen

Helen, age 53, developed an acute skin condition called erythema nodosum at age 30. A large, red, irritated area appeared on one of her legs. She was hospitalized and given intravenous antibiotics and corticosteroids. Shortly after she was discharged from the hospital, she began to feel pain in her joints. This pain, diagnosed as arthritis, plagued her for more than twenty years. It was only when she sought homeopathic care that her arthritis was considerably relieved. As her joint pains improved, Helen briefly re-experienced a rash similar to erythema nodusum on her face and hands. The rash went away and so did her joint pains.

The phenomenon of suppression has been observed by homeopaths since the time of Hahnemann and has become much more prevalent due to the increasing strength of pharmaceuticals and widespread self-treatment with topical hydrocortisone preparations. Whether or not a treatment will be suppressive depends on your state of health, the strength of your resistance to disease, and the intensity and duration of the treatment.

Another common way that suppression occurs is through the use of products such as antiperspirants and antihistamines. Discharges are the body's way to vent waste and the products of disease. In certain susceptible individuals, suppressing a discharge will lead to more serious health problems.

Jamie

Jamie, age 9, was brought to us by his parents because of left hip pain which caused him to limp. He had received conventional care, even hip surgery, without relief. He was a sensitive and delicate child and fit the picture of the homeopathic medicine, *Silica* (flint). Soon after receiving the medicine, the hip pain quickly resolved. We did not see Jamie again for two years. At that time, his parents brought him back for another visit. His hip pain had been completely gone until the previous few weeks, then suddenly returned for no apparent reason. When we questioned Jamie thoroughly, he told us that he had begun to have body odor recently and that his mother had bought him an antiperspirant. Soon after he started using it, his hip pain returned. Patients needing *Silica* are particularly susceptible to illness from suppressed perspiration. He stopped using the antiperspirant, we repeated the *Silica,* and his hip pain again went away quickly.

Your body, in its attempt to keep your symptoms at the most superficial level possible, frequently develops skin eruptions as its first defense. Infants may develop eczema, either at birth or when they are first introduced to cow's milk or formula. If the cow's milk is removed or the child is treated homeopathically, the eczema will usually resolve readily. If the child's eczema is treated with hydro-cortisone cream, the eruption and itch disappear, but the allergic tendency remains. Homeopaths have observed that infants treated in this way may go on to develop asthma, a more serious allergic condition. Although the eczema is gone, the child is much less healthy. If suppression continues, with more hydrocortisone being given to suppress the asthma, then a deeper mental and emotional problem, such as severe depression, may eventually occur.

The body has a reason for generating particular symptoms as part of its attempt to cure the illness. Some medical doctors are beginning to recognize this phenomenon of suppression in childhood asthma. In a study published in the medical journal *Pediatrics* in 1991, the authors speculated that a type of paralysis in asthmatic children may in fact be due to suppression by asthma medications such as steroids.[2]

Hering's Law of Cure

One of the guiding principles in homeopathy is *Hering's law of cure*, named after Constantine Hering, an early American homeopath of German origin. Hering's law states that cure proceeds from top to bottom, from inside out, from most important organs to least important organs, and from most recent to oldest symptoms. Although every case does not follow this order, many cases do, and these principles are often useful in determining whether the remedy is working properly. The idea behind Hering's Law is that your body is always trying to keep symptoms at the most superficial level possible and to promote your overall health, function, and freedom of action. Your defense mechanism will attempt to heal and balance first those structures and functions that have the greatest impact on your health and well-being.

Mary

Mary suffered from eczema during most of her life. For years she had used topical hydrocortisone to control the itching, burning rash that covered her face, neck, torso and arms. The eczema was worse in the bends of her joints and the creases in her skin. Her skin was aggravated by bathing and perspiration. Mary stopped the hydrocortisone before taking her homeopathic medicine. In response to the remedy and discontinuing the hydrocortisone, Mary's eczema came out fiercely. The outbreak lasted for ten days. Mary was given a mild moisturizing cream made from marigold flowers to soothe, but not suppress, the eruption.

Then the rash started to clear from the top down. It left her face and moved down to her neck. Then it began to clear from her torso and became worse on her arms. As the rash on her arms became much worse, the symptoms on the neck and trunk began to clear up. The eczema finally moved down the arms to the hands. As her hands became worse, her arms started to become less itchy. Slowly, over six months, the eczema finished clearing from her body and did not return.

Often mental and emotional symptoms, which occur at a deeper level than physical symptoms, will be alleviated first. In fact, the physical symptoms, such as a skin eruption or a nasal or vaginal discharge may temporarily become worse. When this occurs, it is important to be patient instead of attempting to eliminate the physical problem.

Susan

Susan responded very well to the remedy *Lachesis* for a left ovarian cyst. She did not need the surgery that had been recommended prior to homeopathic treatment. Several months after her cyst disappeared, a rash developed on her face and on the skin just over both ovaries. Despite her discomfort from itching and swelling, she resisted her friend's advice to consult with a dermatologist. Her intuition told her that it was important that she not suppress the rash. She understood that suppressing the rash could result in the return of her cyst. Her homeopath confirmed her intuition and told her that it was best to wait, and that the rash would disappear in time, which it did.

How Is Homeopathy Different From Conventional Medicine?

Homeopathic medicine is based on entirely different concepts than conventional Western medicine. Conventional medicine uses synthetic drugs. Homeopathy uses only natural medicines based on the law of similars.

Conventional medicine aims to destroy bacteria and viruses, control physiological processes, and maintain body functions within the range necessary to sustain life. Homeopathy believes that all these goals can be accomplished by strengthening the individual's resistance and healing abilities. Conventional medicine specializes in understanding the functions and illnesses of discrete parts of the body. Homeopathy specializes in treating the whole person.

Conventional physicians often give many different medicines at one time, each to control a different organ or physiologic process. Homeopaths give only one medicine at a time. *Allopathic* (non-homeopathic) drugs may have serious side effects. Homeopathic medicines may produce additional symptoms during the course of treatment, but these are rarely serious or harmful. Conventional medicine evaluates its rate of success based on whether the immediate condition resolves. Homeopathy attempts to eliminate not only the immediate condition, but also the underlying susceptibility, and to promote long-term health.

Notes

[1] Hahnemann S., *Organon of Medicine.* Sixth Edition, Los Angeles: J. P. Tarcher, 1982, pg. 10.

[2] Shahar, E, Hwang, P, Niesen, C, Murphy, E, "Poliomyelitis-like Paralysis During Recovery from Acute Bronchial Asthma: Possible Etiology and Risk Factors." *Ped* 1991; 88: 276-279.

"Homeopathy cures a larger percentage of cases than any other form of treatment."

— *Mahatma Gandhi.*

WHY CHOOSE
HOMEOPATHY?

Homeopathy is Highly Effective

In acute and chronic disease, whether the symptoms are physical, mental, or emotional, homeopathy produces subtle, yet often dramatic, healing. From newborns to centenarians, most people can benefit from homeopathy. Homeopaths treat common illnesses such as allergies, asthma, digestive disorders, gynecologic problems, skin conditions, insomnia, chronic fatigue, headaches, and arthritis. If the homeopath can find the simillimum for the individual, most diseases with reversible pathology can be treated. Even chronic autoimmune or hereditary diseases such as diabetes, scleroderma, psoriasis, and systemic lupus erythematosis may respond to homeopathic treatment, especially in the early stages of the disease.

Although homeopaths prescribe for the whole person rather than the specific disease state, injuries and acute illnesses, such as colds, flus, fevers, sore throats, and bronchitis can improve very quickly with homeopathic treatment. Homeopaths know that antibiotics are not the only successful treatment for infections. Ear infections, conjunctivitis, bladder infections, vaginal infections, boils, and cellulitis frequently respond well to homeopathic treatment. Many people have come to respect homeopathy after witnessing its rapid action on a painful sore throat or the relief provided by the homeopathic medicine *Arnica montana* (Leopard's bane) after an injury.

In cases of kidney stones, gall bladder disease, ovarian cysts, and uterine fibroids, the need for surgery may sometimes be avoided with prompt homeopathic treatment. In more advanced or emergency cases, surgery may be the treatment of choice. Even when the body is unable to heal the problem completely, the symptoms of these illnesses, such as bleeding, inflammation, and pain, can often be significantly improved. When surgery is necessary, homeopathic medicines such as *Arnica* can help prevent excessive bleeding and speed healing after surgery.

Homeopathy can often provide benefit to patients with neurologic conditions such as Bell's palsy (a type of facial paralysis), epilepsy, carpal tunnel syndrome, twitches, numbness, and sciatica, and other kinds of nerve pain. It may sometimes help multiple sclerosis, Parkinsonism, and other more serious neurologic diseases.

Even homeopaths are sometimes surprised at what homeopathy can accomplish, as in the following case:

Elizabeth

Elizabeth, a 2½ year old girl was diagnosed with cerebral palsy, spastic quadriplegia, blindness, deafness, and microencephaly (a congenitally small head). Her mother had taken drugs throughout her pregnancy. Elizabeth had been malnourished up to the age of two, being fed only 2% milk and weighing only nineteen pounds. Elizabeth was "in her own world". She plugged her ears with her fingers and rolled her head from side to side. Her eyeballs moved in different directions. She hated being touched or bathed and was terrified of having her diaper changed.

Elizabeth could not walk, crawl, or sit, and was able to make only spastic movements of her arms. She never stopped moving her arms unless she was asleep. She slammed her head against the mattress to fall asleep. Her homeopath had no idea how much improvement was possible, but he studied the case and prescribed *Tarentula hispanica.* (Spanish spider). When there was no improvement after five weeks, it was evident that the first remedy was incorrect. He restudied the child's symptoms carefully and then prescribed *Stramonium.* Five weeks later her mother called him to communicate the changes. Elizabeth no longer minded being touched. She loved to play with water now, though she still screamed when she was bathed. She had begun to crawl. She was no longer slamming her head against the mattress. She was still unable to get into a sitting position or to bend her torso.

Three days later her mother reported that Elizabeth had crawled five feet across the living room floor! Four months later she was making some vocal sounds and could crawl on her stomach using her arms. Nine months after being given the correct homeopathic remedy, Elizabeth no longer carried the diagnosis of microencephaly. Her head size was now just over normal. Nor was she still categorized as having cerebral palsy or quadriplegia. She had the full use of her arms and had been actively crawling for seven weeks. She was still blind and had a 70 percent hearing impairment. She was able to hold her head up and sit in a high chair. She continued to be mildly retarded and a year and a half later was doing well in a special education class in the public school system.

Opponents of homeopathy often suggest that its effectiveness has not been scientifically proven in double blind studies, but this is not so. In a 1991 review article in the *British Medical Journal*, a group of Dutch researchers evaluated 107 controlled clinical research studies on homeopathy that had been published in medical journals between 1966 and 1990.[1] Eighty one of the studies showed positive results (76 percent) in such conditions as respiratory and other infections, digestive disorders, influenza, hay fever, recovery after surgery, rheumatoid arthritis, fibromyalgia, and psychological problems. Although the authors of the article thought that some of the research methodology was flawed, in the studies which they rated best, fifteen out of twenty-two (68 percent) still showed positive results.

Homeopathy for Cancer and AIDS

Homeopathic journals from the nineteenth century record cases of cancer treated effectively with homeopathy[2], however no modern studies have been conducted. The medico-legal environment makes cancer treatment a perilous proposition for the practitioner. Some cancer patients seek out homeopathic treatment in addition to surgery, chemotherapy and radiation. In such cases, homeopathy serves to reduce the side effects of the allopathic treatments and to stimulate the body to relieve pain and to promote healing to the greatest extent possible.

Homeopaths treat people who are HIV-positive and have also treated patients with AIDS. Michael Strange, a homeopath in London, has treated seventy HIV-positive patients, sixteen of whom have been under treatment for two to four years. None has gone on to develop symptoms of AIDS. In addition, he had had some success in treating patients who have AIDS. During 1990, only five out of fifty of his patients died of the disease.[3]

In cases of HIV infection, patients under homeopathic treatment are sometimes able to maintain their health and energy and delay progression to AIDS. In a study at Bastyr University in Seattle, HIV-positive patients who received natural therapies, including homeopathy, increased their survival rate and their quality of life as compared with patients receiving conventional treatment alone.[4] Since few AIDS patients have chosen to use homeopathy as their only form of therapy, effectiveness has been difficult to evaluate.

Homeopathy For Mental And Emotional Problems

Homeopathy has the potential for producing far more than just improvements in your physical health. The homeopathic remedy can be a catalyst that starts a process of transformation in your life. Homeopathic medicine can be very successful in treating anxiety, depression, grief, phobias, and other mental disorders. Deeper psychiatric disorders such as autism, the behavioral problems associated with developmental disabilities and schizophrenia have a more guarded prognosis, but can sometimes be helped. Facilities do not yet exist to treat severe mental and emotional problems homeopathically in a safe and controlled environment. Experienced homeopaths may take on some of these cases on an outpatient basis, especially if there is enough support for the patient in her home environment. During the nineteenth century, homeopathic mental hospitals flourished and provided some of the most humane and effective treatment available for mental patients.

John

One night, nearly ten years ago, a patient called a homeopathic practitioner in a panic. She had broken up with her boyfriend, John and he had lost his job the same day. He disappeared, leaving her a suicide note. In the note he said that his life was a failure and he was going to jump off a bridge. She was about to leave to search for him and wanted to know if there was anything that could be prescribed to help him out of his desperate state. The homeopath suggested the remedy *Aurum metallicum*, made from gold. This medicine is for people who feel a deep sense of failure and depression, and who often wish to commit suicide to escape from a life which they perceive to be bleak and hopeless. She notified the police and they found him on the bridge, contemplating his leap. Luckily they arrived just in time to save him. They brought him back and he was cowering in a corner. She gave him a dose of *Aurum*. Within a few hours he no longer felt suicidal. He continued with homeopathic treatment and became a successful architect.

Rosa

Rosa, a 50 year old Mexican woman, complained of terrible anxiety. She had become extremely anxious two years before when her husband suffered a heart attack. She was terrified that he would die. Since that time she was afraid to go anywhere without him, even though he encouraged her to do so. She abandoned all of the activities that she previously enjoyed. She was always afraid that she was doing something wrong. She knew her fears were irrational, but that did not make the situation any better. She had tried anti-anxiety medications without benefit. She was given *Phosphorus*. She has now resumed tennis and engagements with friends. She feels much better about herself, can go on long trips without fear, and is planning a trip to Mexico.

Homeopaths are quite successful in treating children diagnosed with attention deficit disorder and related behavioral disorders. These children often manifest unusual and unique symptoms, which allows the homeopath to more easily find the correct remedy.

Sharon

Sharon, age 16, was referred to a homeopath by her family practice physician because of a five year history of attention deficit disorder. She remembered being sent out of the classroom in kindergarten for talking too much. She had been on stimulant medication since the sixth grade. Sharon hated taking it. She didn't feel like herself, even while on the medicine. Without the medication, Sharon was unable to focus, or pay attention. She became distracted easily by noise or movement, which made it hard for her to take tests in school. When talking to someone, her eyes became tired and she stared into space. She complained of talking without thinking. She told herself to be quiet, but blurted out her thoughts or feelings anyway. She couldn't stop herself. It was sometimes embarrassing to her, though much of the time she had little, if any, self awareness about how she acted with other people. She was unaware of how loudly she spoke and people around her would say "shhh...."

Sharon was always fidgeting and fiddling. She constantly clicked her nails on her teeth or tapped her fingers. She poked, hugged, and pulled at other people, annoying them. She couldn't keep her hands to herself and was always moving some part of her body. "It's not me that's doing these things," she said. "I wouldn't ever be touchy or pokey." Sharon often acted childishly.

At times Sharon felt so hyperactive that she was always moving her fingers, bouncing her knee, or skipping down the hall to release the pent up energy. She had so much energy inside that she felt like screaming. She described it as feeling frustrated and out of control, "as if the energy is trapped and has to be pushed out."

Sharon described herself as "a major procrastinator," regardless of whether she was on medication or not. She was gullible and asked "dumb questions," even though she was very bright and had a 3.8 grade point average. Often the answers just didn't click. She was slow to get a joke.

Her fingers and toes were always cold when she skied. Sharon loved pickles and ate them straight from the jar. She used to eat a lot of salt and lemons. She also liked to suck on ice.

Sharon discontinued the stimulant medication and took *Veratrum album* (white hellebore) and returned in five weeks. She was doing extremely well. Her test grades were improving. The last time she had tried to stop taking the medicine, she had gotten all F's. She remarked that she had found our parking lot without directions, something she could normally do only while on the stimulant medication. Her parents reported that her energy was much more positive. She no longer stared blankly. Her friends told her that she "wasn't as crazy as she used to be." She was not as fidgety anymore and felt a lot more controlled. She now had "a real appetite" instead of just sporadic urges. She was no longer poking, hugging, and pulling other people. Her leg wasn't restless anymore and she had stopped clicking her nails against her teeth. She didn't have "that special taste" for pickles anymore, but she was still thirsty and procrastinated just as much.

Sharon was given another dose of the *Veratrum* three months later after eating coffee-flavored candy that interfered with the remedy. A year later, she continued to do remarkably well. She began to experience some sensations and tastes that she had not had since she was a little girl. She was no longer staring into space. She noticed when she became hyperactive and could stop it, which she had been unable to do before the homeopathy. "It's like somebody opened the curtains and let me see." She was now able to notice when her voice got loud and quieted down. She became fidgety only once in a while. Sharon was a changed young woman.

As you experience the benefits of homeopathic treatment, you are likely to experience more energy, to have a clearer mind, a sharper memory, and more balanced emotions. After being given a remedy, homeopathic patients often report, "I feel like myself again." You may not even notice all the changes in yourself at first, but others will. They may ask, "What did you do for yourself? You seem so happy and healthy!" You may also respond differently to others. You may find that you are more tolerant with people who used to irritate you. You may also find yourself standing up to someone who used to dominate you.

Sometimes these changes take some getting used to. Your relationships may shift as your internal patterns change. You may find yourself being less dependent on others as your health improves and this can be disconcerting to those who have been your caregivers. You are likely to be stronger and more resilient. It is good to let the people around you know that you are going through a healing process, that they can expect you to be different, and that you might be making some changes in your life that may surprise them.

Homeopathy and psychotherapy often work well together. This combination of therapies is especially important in people who have been sexually abused or have experienced other types of trauma and need extensive help to process these experiences. Patients with anorexia or bulimia or with chemical dependencies also benefit most from using both therapies. Homeopathic treatment can speed the process of psychotherapy by allowing the patient to access deeper issues more quickly. Patients often make psychological breakthroughs using homeopathy and subsequently decide to begin psychotherapy to explore their issues on a deeper level. Psychotherapy allows people to process the feelings that come up as they become healthier emotionally during the homeopathic process. Psychotherapy also helps patients integrate into their lives the changes that result from homeopathic treatment.

Callie

Callie, age 35, came from an abusive, alcoholic home. Her parents always told her that she was ugly and couldn't do anything right. She eventually believed them. She went from one oppressive and demeaning job and relationship to another. By the time she consulted a homeopath, she was suicidally depressed and very angry. She hated her boss. She didn't have the courage to stand up to him to his face, but she would go home and swear at him at the top of her lungs. A combination of treatment with homeopathic *Anacardium* (marking nut) and intensive work with a psychotherapist helped to relieve her suicidal feelings and allow her to feel more positive about her own abilities. At this time, she is still working for the same boss, but realizes that it is only a matter of time before she will move on to a job that better suits her.

Ashley

Ashley, a 37 year old kindergarten teacher, was referred for homeopathic treatment by her psychotherapist because of depression, profuse menstrual bleeding, chronic muscle pain, and a history of sexual abuse. She complained to her homeopath of a painful whiplash injury which occurred during a recent car accident. When questioned further, Ashley recounted a history of a series of car accidents. Hearing the history of accidents and noticing the broken blood vessel in Ashley's right eye, her homeopath began to consider the homeopathic remedy *Arnica montana*, mentioned previously as a major remedy for trauma, whiplash, bruising, bleeding and muscle soreness.

Ashley shared that each time her sexual abuser had assaulted her, he would push her down on the ground. She would feel extremely sore and bruised the following day. Knowing that an individual's pattern or story frequently reflects itself in dreams, her homeopath inquired about any recurrent dreams. Ashley dreamed repeatedly of being a frog jumping from one lily pad to the next. Despite the soft surface of the lily pads, wherever she landed, she would feel sore and bruised. She also dreamed of car accidents.

In an effort to understand the origin of this theme of injury, the homeopath inquired as to any trauma during birth or in utero. Ashley reported that she was given a transfusion at birth, at which time she was separated from her mother.

After receiving *Arnica*, not only did Ashley's muscle pain, heavy menstrual bleeding, and depression improve, but her dreams changed. She dreamed that she backed up her car in a parking lot. Another car backed up at the same time and they almost hit, but they didn't. She thought this was curious because in her past dreams the two cars would collide. The next day, Ashley reported, this very incident occurred in real life and an accident was avoided. This is the level of reprogramming that is possible with homeopathy.

The homeopath then inquired as to whether Ashley's mother experienced any traumas or accidents during her pregnancy with Ashley. Ashley didn't know at the time, but called back the next day after speaking with her mother. When her mother was four or five months pregnant with her, she and her husband were on the way to an appointment with the obstetrician when a trailer truck pulled out and headed straight towards them. The only way they could avoid an accident was for her husband to immediately veer off the road. It was a frightening experience for both of them and may have initiated the theme of accidents and trauma in Ashley's life.

Homeopathy for Animals

Opponents of homeopathy say that homeopathic medicines act only as a placebo, but if this were true, why would animals respond so well to homeopathic treatment? A number of homeopathy books have been written by veterinarians, of whom a small, but growing, number now incorporate homeopathy into their practices.

We have found excellent success in treating our own animals with homeopathy over the past ten years.

Jasmine and Leila Rose

Our six month old golden retriever puppy, Jasmine, began to limp after we took her jogging for a couple of days. The veterinarian diagnosed her condition as osteochondritis dessicans, an inflammation of the cartilage. The veterinarian recommended that she be given no exercise for a few weeks and that surgery would probably be needed. We treated her with *Calcarea phosphorica*, a well known remedy for bone and cartilage problems. Several days later she was bouncing around like her exuberant puppy self. Now, three years later, she jogs with us regularly and has had no further problems.

We also have a 13 year old golden retriever named Leila Rose. Each time she went backpacking with us, she would lie in every icy, cold stream she could find. We would wake the next morning in our tent to find Leila stiff and shivering. By the time we got home, she could barely jump out of our station wagon. She would limp inside the door and fall into a heap. She was so stiff and sore that she could not even walk up the stairs to her dinner. She would just lie limp and shivering. This first happened when she was six years old. We were very frightened that she might die. We took her to a veterinary emergency room. They didn't know what was wrong with her. We thought about what caused this state and realized it was a combination of her exposure to the cold streams and overexertion. We gave her homeopathic *Rhus toxicodendron* and she was back to her playful self within hours. Leila has continued to benefit from *Rhus toxicodendron* for the past seven years.

Homeopathy Is Safe

Homeopathy is one of the safest forms of medicine, even for pregnant women, infants, and the elderly. Any toxic effects of a crude substance in nature disappear when that substance is prepared homeopathically. In order for it to be made into a homeopathic medicine, the substance is diluted sufficiently to eliminate all toxic effects.

Because it tastes like candy, many children have swallowed an entire bottle of homeopathic medicine, with no ill effects. Homeopathic medicines do not cause allergic reactions. If a person repeatedly takes a specific homeopathic medicine that is not appropriate for him or her, it is possible for that individual to begin to experience some new symptoms, called *proving symptoms,* but this rarely occurs when a patient is treated by an experienced prescriber. When proving symptoms do occur, they are generally mild and usually disappear when the medicine is stopped. Homeopathic medicines are recognized by the United States Food and Drug Administration to be so safe that most are classified as over the counter medicines.

Homeopathy is Cost Effective

Unlike pharmaceutical drugs, homeopathic medicines are very inexpensive. Enough homeopathic medicine to last several months or years is likely to cost less than a single course of antibiotics. The main cost of homeopathy is the office visit. Many people consider homeopathic treatment a bargain when compared with the other available treatment options. Homeopathy may prevent future hospitalizations by keeping you in good health, resulting in substantial long-term savings. Patient visits are generally infrequent compared to conventional medicine, acupuncture, and chiropractic care.

Insurance reimbursement for homeopathy depends on the terms of your policy and the license of your practitioner. If your company does not cover your homeopathic practitioner, you may wish to request that the coverage be added to your policy or consider switching insurance companies. Even if homeopathic treatment is not covered by your insurance, many patients find that it is well worth the additional expense.

Blue Cross of Washington and Alaska set up a series of town meetings throughout the state of Washington to find out what type of medical treatment people wanted. A large number of people attending these meetings strongly expressed their desire to have homeopathic medicine covered by their insurance, which led Blue Cross of Washington to establish, in 1994, their Alternapath pilot program covering homeopathy, naturopathy, and acupuncture. Hopefully other companies will follow suit.

Homeopathy Can Enhance the Effects of Conventional Medicine

When conventional medicine is necessary, homeopathy can still be of great benefit. If you take the remedy *Arnica* before and after surgery, your healing process will generally be much faster. We have seen this repeatedly with many types of surgery, including dental surgery, repair of fractures, hysterectomies, and plastic surgery. Surgeons are often surprised that their patients who use homeopathy need little or no pain medication after surgery and recover quickly. Homeopathy can often relieve the nausea which results as a side effect from chemotherapy. In cases of terminal illness, homeopathic remedies may ease the transition into death.

Madeline

Robert was able to attend his mother at her bedside during the last month of her life as she was dying from lung cancer. Although the cancer had metastasized and it was no longer possible to prevent her death, her suffering was considerably relieved. One of her main problems, towards the end, was difficulty in breathing due to mucus congestion in her lungs. She had been prescribed morphine and scopalamine patches to ease her breathing. The morphine made her drowsy and the scopalamine caused confusion and hallucinations. Robert prescribed the homeopathic medicine *Carbo vegetabilis* (charcoal) which helped her breathe more easily, making the other medications unnecessary. She was able to die peacefully at home, surrounded by her family, free of pain, and was lucid until just before she died.

Notes

1 Kleijnan J, Knipschild, P, ter Riet G. "Clinical Trials of Homeopathy." *Brit Med J* 1991; 302:316-323.

2 Murphy R., *Homeopathic Medicine and Cancer,* Portland: Murphy, 1983.

3 Ullman, D., Address to the California Homeopathic Medical Society, April 21, 1992.

4 Standish L, Guiltanan J, McMahon E, Lindstrom, C., "One Year Open Trial of Naturopathic Treatment of HIV Infection Class IV-A in Men." *J Naturopathic Med*, 1992; 3:42-64.

"Poisons kill.
Poisons cure.
It depends on how
you use them."

— *Indian sage.*

From Snake Venom to Squid Ink

The Source of Homeopathic Medicines

Homeopathic remedies are derived from substances ranging from the exotic to the mundane. The material for homeopathic remedies is collected from plants, animals, and minerals from all over the world. Everything in the natural world is fair game when it comes to making homeopathic medicines and will act curatively if the symptoms that it causes in a healthy person match those of the person being treated.

Nux vomica, a remedy for ambitious, hard driving, workaholic people with spasmodic symptoms, irritability and sleeplessness, comes from a plant from the Phillippines known as Quaker's buttons or poison nut. *Arnica montana*, for bruises, sprained ankles and traumatic injuries, comes from a pretty yellow flower that grows in the mountains, where such injuries are likely to occur. *Sepia* is primarily a remedy for women who are feeling depressed, irritable, weepy, and have lost their sex drive. They may suffer from morning sickness, hot flashes, or menstrual or liver problems. Patients needing *Sepia* generally feel much better after vigorous exercise. *Sepia* comes from squid ink, which was used in quill pens over a century ago. Women who repeatedly licked the quills to moisten their pens developed these symptoms. Men also may occasionally need *Sepia*.

Ted

Ted sought help for a chronic hepatitis that drained him of his energy. He was a triathlete, but his fatigue left him unable to compete, even though he found exercise exhilarating. Ted was skinny, sallow, and looked very sad. During the course of the first homeopathic interview, Ted revealed that his symptoms had begun while he was working as a prep cook in a natural foods restaurant. His job, each day, was to cut up hundreds of squid to be served as a macrobiotic delicacy. The more he handled the squid, the sicker he became. His direct contact with the squid, along with his specific symptoms, led us to prescribe *Sepia*. This remedy helped him to regain his stamina and he was once again entering triathalons.

Other remedies are made from very common substances, such as table salt, coffee beans, sand, oyster shells, and metals including iron, copper, aluminum, and gold. A few currently used allopathic medicines are made from these same substances. Gold shots, for example, may be used for difficult cases of rheumatoid arthritis. Platinum is the main constituent of a widely used drug for cancer treatment.

Poisons as Medicine

Even extremely poisonous substances such as the venom of the Bushmaster snake (*Lachesis*), become nontoxic when prepared homeopathically.

Natalie

Natalie, pregnant for the first time at age 33, sought out a homeopath for severe varicose veins of her left leg when she was seven months pregnant. At the suggestion of her obstetrician, she was wearing support hose all the time, but felt no relief. She was miserable. What bothered her the most was the severe throbbing and aching of her leg, which was worse from standing for even a short time. Six days after she received *Lachesis*, the pain was completely gone. She no longer wore support hose except when she needed to stand all day. She enjoyed the remainder of her pregnancy and delivered a healthy little girl.

Thorn apple (*Datura stramonium*), a poisonous plant, is the source of the homeopathic medicine *Stramonium* and is known to treat patients suffering from hallucinations, rage, violence, nightmares, and strong fears of the dark or water. This remedy, due to the strongly violent nature of contemporary American culture and media, is prescribed with great frequency by modern homeopaths.

Mark

Mark, age 5, was brought in by his mother because of his violent and abusive behavior. He screamed, scratched, cursed, threw things at people, and bit people, all of which seemed to be out of his conscious control. He once pounded a developmentally disabled child in the face. His mother described his personality as Dr. Jekyll and Mr. Hyde. When asked what he most liked to do, Mark responded, "Kill dinosaurs." This child cursed when he was angry, which happened every day. Mark also had facial tics, tongue clicking, and grimaces. After being given *Stramonium*, Mark's tics and grimaces disappeared within one month. He completely stopped cursing and had only rare angry outbursts, with none of the previous violence and intensity.

Who can forget the red, itching blistering eruptions of poison ivy? Known as *Rhus toxicodendron*, poison ivy is an excellent medicine for skin eruptions, arthritis, injuries, and ailments from overexertion. Called the "rusty gate remedy," it relieves joint stiffness and pain that develops after exposure to cold, damp weather or cold water.

Arsenicum album, made from arsenic, is one of the best remedies for anxiety and insomnia. People who have been poisoned with arsenic become extremely restless, chilly, agitated, and terrified of death. Homeopathic *Arsenicum album* can bring great relief to a person in such a state of anxiety.

Evelyn

Evelyn, 64 years old, was in a terrible state. She had been suffering from tremendous anxiety with a racing heart, feelings of panic, and a tremendous fear of being alone, which was quite unlike her usual independent self. She woke at three in the morning with a dry mouth worrying about who would take care of her if she became ill. She feared that she would be taken to a mental hospital or have a heart attack or a stroke. She felt very jittery and had developed a nervous stomach. She vacillated between feeling very hot, with needle-like sensations, to having "nervous chills." *Arsenicum album* relieved her of the anxiety and allowed her to "feel like herself again."

Salts of the Earth

Many minerals have found their way into the homeopathic materia medica. The most common of these is table salt, known as *Natrum muriaticum*. It is a useful medicine for headaches, cold sores, sinusitis, allergies, and conditions in which the person feels worse from being out in the sun. People needing this remedy are extremely sensitive and get their feelings hurt easily. They isolate themselves and cry their salty tears only in solitude.

Karen

Karen's chief complaints were a rash around her mouth and recurrent genital herpes. She was a very sensitive woman who had experienced grief due to an unhappy childhood. When asked about her food cravings, she said she loved salty foods like potato chips. After taking *Natrum muriaticum,* her skin rashes were gone, and her herpes outbreaks were few and far between. It is interesting to note that this woman was a musician, because people needing *Natrum muriaticum* are known to be very deeply affected by music.

Kali carbonicum (potassium carbonate), is a useful medicine for joint pain, asthma, and gas. Patients needing this remedy often complain of a feeling of anxiety in their stomach. They commonly wake at night between two and four a.m.

Doris

While on vacation, Doris developed an acute sciatica that woke her up at three a.m. every night. The only way she could relieve her pain was to get up and walk around. *Kali carbonicum* relieved the pain considerably and allowed Doris to enjoy the rest of her travels.

From Dog's Milk to Red Ants

Animal substances make an important contribution to the homeopathic materia medica. We have already mentioned honeybee and squid ink. Dog's milk (*Lac caninum*) is helpful for breast problems of nursing mothers. It is also useful for some people with low self-esteem, a disconnected or floating sensation, and symptoms that alternate sides.

Ginny

Ginny, age 38, suffered the devastating loss of her infant daughter due to sudden infant death syndrome. Her breast milk continued to flow, continually reminding her of the loss of her precious child. When we gave her *Lac caninum,* her breast milk quickly dried up within a few days. Ginny went on to have a healthy son.

Red ants *(Formica rufa)* are used for wandering arthritic pains and for eruptions that look like ant bites. An article in the Seattle Post-Intelligencer began by saying, "A handful of ants a day keeps the doctor away." The article explained that ants had been found to be especially effective against rheumatism, according to the Chinese entomological society, because of the formic acid in the insects. More than 250,000 rheumatism sufferers had been successfully treated by using ant remedies. Ants wander and bite. What they cause, they can cure.

*Theridion (*the Orange spider), is good for anyone who has a tremendous sensitivity to noise, which seems to go right through them, especially into the teeth, causing nausea and dizziness.

Danny

Danny, a 5 year old boy, was brought for homeopathic care by his mother because of his insomnia. He would wake in the middle of the night with great fear and crawl into his parents' bed. When asked what he was afraid of, he replied that it was the noises outside the house that scared him and woke him up. He would always cover his ears when he heard loud noises and had a frequent habit of making nervous grimaces. After being treated with *Theridion,* Danny was able to sleep through the night and was no longer fearful of noises. His nervous system was calmed and the grimaces disappeared.

The Homeopathic Healing Power of Plants

One of the most important sources of homeopathic medicine is the plant kingdom. Chamomile tea *(Chamomilla)*, a common herbal beverage, is the friend of many a mother with a cranky, irritable child who is in great pain from teething or an earache.

Johnny

Johnny's mom was at her wit's end with her 18 month old son because nothing pleased him. He had a tough kid look on his face, pushed other kids who were in his way, and always seemed to wake up grumpy. Johnny suffered from chronic ear infections and the doctors were recommending myringotomy tubes. His parents remembered that homeopathic *Chamomilla* had helped him in the past with his teething. After another dose of *Chamomilla,* he was much easier to live with again and his ear infections improved dramatically.

Pulsatilla, the wind flower, is highly effective in many cases of gentle, tearful women with menstrual difficulties or irregularities. It is also used for people who are suffering from a "ripe" cold with profuse yellow nasal discharge. People needing *Pulsatilla* often feel too hot and love the open air. They are usually not very thirsty.

Susie

Susie tried homeopathy because of her mood swings and depression. She had recently remembered a history of sexual abuse as a child and felt very sad and angry. She was plump and had the appearance of a little girl, even though she was in her late thirties. She talked about her fear of abandonment, which began when she was very young. Susie's periods were painful and irregular. She had lots of gas, especially when she ate fried foods or meat. *Pulsatilla* helped Susie to feel much stronger within herself. Her mood swings and weepiness improved, her menstrual cycle became regular, and she could handle fried foods without indigestion,

New Remedies

Even though the number of remedies is already large, new ones are still being discovered. New remedies are being added to information on homeopathic remedies, called the *materia medica,* as they are proven. Recent provings of *Hydrogen*, *Chocolate*, and *Scorpion* have been conducted by a British homeopath, Jeremy Sherr. People taking *Hydrogen* experienced a great feeling of lightness and exhilaration followed by a profound sense of disconnectedness. *Chocolate*, in its homeopathic form, is useful for certain people who have strong emotional feelings about mothering and being nurtured. These people often have a strong craving for chocolate. One woman in his study ate two pounds of chocolate a day! Those proving *Scorpion* developed tendencies of maliciousness and antisocial behavior and felt most comfortable in isolation.

The more homeopathic
remedies are
diluted and shaken,
the stronger their
action becomes.

THE UNIQUE PREPARATION OF HOMEOPATHIC MEDICINES

The Homeopathic Paradox: Weaker Is Stronger

Homeopathic remedies are prepared by a process of serial dilution and shaking known as *potentization*. The more homeopathic remedies are diluted and shaken, the stronger their action becomes. Chemically, the substance becomes more and more dilute. Clinically, however, Hahnemann found that the more a substance was potentized, the less often it needed to be given to the patient to produce a curative action and the deeper was its effect. Now, over 150 years after Hahnemann's death, homeopaths continue to validate this observation and cure patients with what seem to be infinitesimally small doses of natural substances.

The degree of dilution of homeopathic remedies may seem extraordinary. Imagine one drop of ink dissolved in ten drops of water. Only 1/10 of the ink would be present. If you diluted it again, only 1/100 of the ink would remain. Barely any color would still be visible. Now, repeat this process until you have made six dilutions. Only one part per *million* of the original drop of ink would remain in the solution, and the mixture would appear colorless. This 6x potency is one of the *least* diluted, or weakest, potencies commonly used in homeopathic practice. Imagine how dilute that drop of ink would be after being diluted one thousand, ten thousand or even one million times!

The popularly held belief, when it comes to medicine, is "more is better." Homeopaths have found just the opposite to be true. It is this concept of using infinitesimal doses that has caused many people, including most proponents of conventional medicine, to reject homeopathy categorically without further investigation. However, it is successful daily clinical experience that allows homeopaths to accept this seemingly paradoxical proposition as true.

Potentization

The dilutions of the original substance are called potencies. There are two commonly used dilution scales, X or *decimal*, and C or *centesimal*. X potencies are diluted 1 to 9 and C potencies are diluted 1 to 99. To make an X potency, 1 part of the original substance is added to 9 parts of solvent. To make a C potency, 1 part of the original substance is added to 99 parts of solvent. The 6C potency is 10 times as dilute as the 6X. The most common potencies prepared by pharmacies in the United States range from 6C (6 dilutions) to CM (100,000 dilutions). Many homeopaths refer to potencies fo 30C or below as *low* potencies and potencies of 200C or above as *high* potencies.

The Importance of Succussion

Shaking each dilution is the crucial factor in preparation. It allows a homeopathic remedy to remain potent past the point where none of the original molecules of the substance remain in the dilution. This vigorous shaking is known as *succussion.* Hahnemann originally succussed each remedy by rapping the vial against a large, leatherbound book. In modern manufacturing, it is performed by machine. Succussion allows the medicinal power of the substance to be enhanced far beyond what is possible with simple dilution. The purely chemical effect of a substance is lost as it is diluted more and more, but the homeopathic effects are released, as long as each dilution is shaken. With succussion, the homeopathic remedy gets stronger and longer lasting with each successive dilution.

Hahnemann came upon the idea of succussion after noticing that the medicines he took with him on house calls were more potent than those he kept in his office. This observation led him to succuss, not just dilute, his homeopathic remedies.

How Homeopathic Medicines Are Dispensed and Sold

Homeopathic remedies are dispensed in the form of pellets, liquid dilutions, or tablets for internal use, and salves, tinctures, and ointments for external use. Your homeopath will either dispense the remedy to you directly or will instruct you to obtain it from a homeopathic pharmacy. Although most homeopaths in the United States give the remedies in the form of pellets or tablets, the remedies may also be given in water.

As long as the correct remedy is given, nearly any mode of administration will produce a positive effect. One homeopathic patient went to her homeopath for help with anxiety and insomnia. The homeopath prescribed *Arsenicum album* to take orally. The patient misunderstood the instructions and dumped the contents of the envelope in her bath water. The remedy still worked.

Many herb and natural food stores and pharmacies stock twenty or thirty single homeopathic remedies, usually in the 6X or 30C potency. Homeopathic pharmacies sometimes restrict the sale of high potency remedies to practitioners only, as their safe use requires adequate training. Kits of low potency remedies for home use are sold by most homeopathic pharmacies.

Homeopathic Dosages

A dose is defined by the frequency of taking the remedy rather than by the amount given. Your homeopath will instruct you how often to take a dose. There are specific guidelines that homeopaths follow in deciding when and how often to administer a particular remedy. If you are being treated by a homeopathic practitioner, it is a good idea to ask her before self-administering any homeopathic medicines, even for minor illnesses. Taking a homeopathic remedy at the wrong time can interfere with the healing process.

Willie

Willie, 9 years old, was being treated successfully for a learning disability and a recurrent cough and rash. His attentiveness and aptitude for learning, as confirmed by his teachers, had improved substantially during the course of a year and a half of homeopathic treatment with the remedy *Baryta carbonica* (barium carbonate). After Willie's mother prescribed several doses of *Rhus toxicodendron* for what she thought to be an outbreak of chicken pox, Willie relapsed within one week and needed another dose of his original remedy. If Willie's mom had called his homeopath before giving him the *Rhus toxicodendron,* an alternative could have been suggested that would have relieved the itching but not interfered with his homeopathic treatment.

Depending on the circumstances of your case, your homeopath may choose to administer the remedy either in a single dose, with a relatively long period of time before repeating the medicine, or in more frequent, perhaps even daily, doses. In other circumstances, a single high potency dose may be given followed by a low potency remedy given daily or at other prescribed intervals. The practitioner may recommend that you continue to take the remedy for a certain time period, or that you stop taking it when you feel better. How often the dose is repeated depends on many factors including the strength of your vital force and whether you are taking allopathic medications. Prescription drugs sometimes interfere with the action of homeopathic medicines and make it necessary for your homeopath to instruct you to take your remedy more frequently. If your vital force is not very strong, or you are very sensitive to medications, the remedy may be given more frequently, but in a lower potency, so as not to aggravate your symptoms unnecessarily.

Combination Remedies

Combination remedies for teething, bedwetting, colds, flus, bladder infections, sinusitis, and other minor illnesses can be useful if you don't have access to a trained homeopath. Combinations contain the most common single remedies for a given condition, with the hope that the single remedy that *you* need will be among those in the combination. For example, a flu remedy might contain *Aconitum napellus, Gelsemium, Bryonia,* and *Eupatorium,* the most prescribed remedies for treating influenza. Teething tablets, produced by most of the homeopathic pharmacies, are one the most effective of the combination remedies. A large number of infants with teething problems need *Chamomilla*, which is one of the remedies included in all of the teething combinations.

Many people report getting relief from combination remedies for minor illnesses, but if you do not benefit from these remedies, it is because the single remedy you need is not contained in the combination. This is the time to see an experienced homeopath. Although combination remedies may be effective in some acute illnesses, they are never recommended for chronic conditions. If taken over time, they can confuse a chronic case and make it difficult for an experienced homeopath to find the correct remedy. Experienced homeopaths find that the greatest and most long lasting improvements in health result from taking the similliumum in the form of a single remedy rather than in combination with other remedies.

Billy

One mother complained to a homeopath that homeopathy didn't work. Her son Billy had a dry, irritating cough. She had purchased a homeopathic combination for coughs that contained *Bryonia, Phosphorus, Drosera, Spongia,* and *Aconite,* all of which are excellent for coughs, but his cough did not improve. When the homeopath asked about the cough, the child said he had a tickle and pointed to the base of his throat. Recognizing this to be a characteristic symptom of the medicine *Rumex,* the homeopath gave it to the child. One dose was all that was needed to alleviate his cough.

Teething Children

Many crying, teething children experience initial relief from a combination teething remedy containing *Chamomilla.* Because combination remedies are low potency, they often need several doses a day to get results. After a few days or weeks, mothers sometimes complain that the combination no longer works. In such cases, the low dose of *Chamomilla* in the combination remedy may have simply exhausted its effectiveness and a higher potency may be needed. When *Chamomilla* is given to these children by itself in a higher potency, the effect may last much longer.

A common complaint among patients of conventional medicine is that their practitioners do not listen to them. You won't be able to say that about your homeopath.

Getting to Know the Patient from the Inside Out

The Homeopathic Consultation

Homeopaths conduct an extensive and careful interview or *case taking* lasting one to two hours on the first visit and approximately thirty minutes on return visits. A common complaint among patients of conventional medicine is that their practitioners do not listen to them. You won't be able to say that about your homeopath.

The purpose of the homeopathic consultation is to understand you as a whole person and how your vital force is expressing itself in the form of symptoms. Your homeopath attempts to understand your unique symptoms. An idiosyncrasy that you might have thought to be irrelevant may be the key your homeopath needs to find the right medicine for you. If you have asthma, you are likely to wheeze and feel tightness in your chest. The fact that *you* only wheeze at the seashore, when you hold a cat, while you are singing, after you drink a beer, or at exactly 2 a.m., makes *your* asthma unique and allows the correct remedy to be found.

Mary

Mary, a 9 year old girl with asthma, found that her wheezing came on after being exposed to cold, damp conditions like skiing or swimming in cold water. The remedy that fit this symptom the best was *Natrum sulphuricum* (sodium sulphate), which rapidly helped her condition. After the remedy she was much more tolerant to cold and damp.

An conventional physician will generally ask you only about your chief complaint. A homeopath views the chief complaint as only the beginning, and wants to know much more about you. He will ask you about your physical symptoms and your emotions. Traumatic incidents from the past that might shed light on your present symptoms are also important. Your medical and family history as well as what you were like as a child are taken into account. You will be asked what was happening in your life at the time your symptoms first appeared, what makes your symptoms better or worse, and under what circumstances they occur. Your homeopath will inquire about your memory and concentration and about your relationships with others. The more accurate the information you provide, the easier it will be for your practitioner to prescribe correctly.

Once you have told your story to the best of your ability, your homeopath begins to see the patterns of possible remedies and will ask you specific questions to confirm the symptoms of certain remedies under consideration for your case. You will be asked which foods you crave and dislike and which ones make you sick; whether you like hot or cold drinks or food; and if you are a chilly or a warm person. Your sleep is important, including insomnia, dreams, favorite position, whether you like the window open or closed, and whether you get hot in bed at night. You may be questioned about how much you perspire and about your sexual desire, whether you like the ocean or the mountains, and what kind of weather makes you feel worse. Just relax and do your best to share what is going on with you. Whatever information you give will be carefully listened to, respected, and held in confidence. Your unique symptoms are crucial to finding the correct homeopathic medicine. The fine lines of difference between remedies make it very important that you tell your homeopath all about yourself.

Your homeopath may perform a physical examination or recommend laboratory testing. Laboratory tests can rule out hidden pathology and serve as a baseline for measuring the progress of your treatment. This is important, for example, in monitoring the size of a uterine fibroid through pelvic ultrasounds or measuring serum thyroid levels in the case of a thyroid disorder. You will find that homeopaths generally order only those laboratory tests that are necessary and that testing is not as primary a source of information as it is for a conventional physician.

The Books of the Homeopath

Books are the tools of the homeopath. You may notice that your homeopath, during the interview, flips through a thick book. This indispensable book is called a repertory and includes nearly every symptom imaginable, followed by a list of all the homeopathic medicines that have been known to cure that particular symptom. The repertory that has been used most universally is *Kent's Repertory*, but some other excellent repertories have been published recently.

The other principal type of book that your homeopath will consult is called a materia medica, consisting of many chapters, each including most of the information known about a particular remedy. The *Materia Medica with Repertory* by Boericke, *Lectures on Homeopathic Materia Medica* by Kent, and *Desktop Guide to Keynotes and Confirmatory Symptoms* by Morrison are widely used, although many other excellent materia medicas are available. These and many other books are now available in comprehensive computer database programs such as MacRepertory, ReferenceWorks, CARA, and RADAR (see Appendix).

*"All these things
must be eliminated
or else avoided as
much as possible
if cure is not to be
prevented or impeded."*

— *Samuel Hahnemann,
Organon of Medicine, Sixth Edition.*

Dos and Don'ts for Homeopathic Patients

Taking the Remedy

After taking your case, your practitioner will select the single homeopathic medicine, or *remedy,* that best matches your symptoms and will either give you the remedy or have you buy it at a homeopathic pharmacy. The remedy is impregnated on grains, pellets or tablets, made of either table sugar (sucrose) or milk sugar (lactose). A dose of remedy is one or more of these grains, pellets or tablets placed on or under the tongue. Unlike most medicine, homeopathic remedies are sweet and pleasant tasting. Your practitioner will instruct you as to exactly how often to take your remedy

Dos and Don'ts About Taking Homeopathic Remedies

While under homeopathic treatment for chronic illness, it is best to notify your homeopath before taking any new medications or other homeopathic remedies. In a first aid or emergency situation, however, you should take the appropriate remedy or action immediately and call your practitioner afterwards.

Avoid touching the remedy with your hands if you have recently handled a strong smelling substance. Use the vial cap or a clean spoon, and place the remedy under your tongue to avoid contaminating the remedy.

Don't expose your remedy to direct sunlight, high temperatures, magnets, electromagnetic fields, or strong aromatic odors such as camphor, solvents, paint, and chemicals.

Antidoting

Certain substances or influences can disturb the vital force, interfering with the action of the homeopathic medicine. This phenomenon is commonly known as *antidoting.* When antidoting occurs, the healing effects of the remedy stop, either temporarily or permanently, and your symptoms return, partially or completely. The relapse is usually sudden, but may be gradual. The cause of antidoting is unknown. It may occur at any point in treatment, in rare cases even two years or more after a remedy has been given. After the healing response to a homeopathic remedy has stabilized, you may be more resistant to antidoting factors.

Debbie

Debbie's health improved dramatically from *Sulphur*. Her vaginal irritation was improved, her hemorrhoids were gone, her premenstrual symptoms were no longer a problem, and her energy was much better. That is, until she ate some coffee-flavored cookies at a Christmas party. "A week later my constipation, hemorrhoids, and vaginal itching returned. I felt dramatically different. After feeling so good for seven months after taking *Sulphur,* my health took a nosedive. My energy lagged. I had headaches, mood swings, and premenstrual acne again. By mid-January, I couldn't stand feeling so bad anymore. I went back to get another remedy. Make sure those cookies don't have espresso in them. It's really not worth it."

Tess

Tess had derived considerable benefit from *Borax* for her joint pains and touchy moods. Many of her symptoms returned less than one month after she took her last homeopathic remedy. Her homeopath was puzzled and decided to wait another month to evaluate Tess' symptoms. As Tess checked out with the clinic receptionist, she took a jar out of her purse. "By the way, I want to make sure this lip balm is compatible with homeopathic remedies. On reading the label, her homeopath noticed that camphor was one of the first ingredients. This explained why her symptoms had returned so soon.

The substances and influences listed below may interfere with the action of homeopathic remedies when a sensitive patient is exposed to them, but the approach taken by each practitioner to the issue of antidoting varies. Practitioners often give their patients a list of substances to avoid, which can be brief or more extensive. Other homeopaths do not make antidoting an issue unless it actually occurs. Some homeopaths believe that antidoting never happens to their patients, and consider other explanations if the remedy does not act as long as expected.

A number of homeopathic practitioners estimate that the treatment of approximately 60 percent of their patients will be adversely affected by ingesting coffee. Your homeopath may recommend that you avoid coffee entirely or she may say nothing at all until she sees whether the treatment has been successful.

The guidelines below are what we give to our patients based on our own clinical experience and a consensus of homeopaths we have consulted. Their opinions varied with their own experience with patients. We have seen many cases in which the substances and influences below have interfered with homeopathic treatment. We prefer to err in the direction of being overcautious, particularly while we are still trying to find the best remedy for the patient. What is most important is that that you follow the instructions of *your* homeopath in this matter.

What to Avoid While Under Homeopathic Treatment

Coffee: This is the one substance that most often interferes with homeopathic treatment. Even one sip of coffee, decaf, or a small amount of coffee in ice cream, liqueur, or candy may be sufficient to disturb the treatment in very sensitive patients. Other patients may need to drink several cups of coffee or drink coffee regularly for a period of time to cause their symptoms to return. In some patients, coffee does not interfere. It appears to be a variety of compounds in coffee rather than just the caffeine that creates the problem. Other caffeinated substances, such as black tea and cola drinks, although not considered healthy, do not usually interfere with homeopathic treatment.

Electric blankets: They can affect the action of remedies by affecting your body's electromagnetic field.

Aromatic substances: Avoid camphor, eucalyptus, and any products that contain them including liniments, lip balms, mouthwashes, cough drops and lozenges. This includes aromatherapy oils and other aromatic compounds such as tea tree products. Strong fumes from oil based paint, turpentine, and paint thinner, certain household cleaning agents containing pine oil or phenol, as well as strong smelling industrial chemicals may also interfere, depending on individual sensitivity.

Medications: Homeopathic medicines will not prevent prescription drugs from working, but some prescription drugs may interfere with homeopathic remedies. In individual cases, topical or oral medications such as antibiotics, narcotics and steroids can interfere. Consult with your practitioner about any drugs that you are taking.

Immunizations: Immunizations sometimes interrupt the homeopathic healing process in certain individuals. Whether you take them or not is your personal choice, but you may want to discuss each specific immunization and your particular circumstances with your homeopath.

Dental work: Dental drilling and the use of novocaine may disturb the effects of homeopathic remedies. It is preferable, if possible, to wait at least three or four months after taking a remedy to have dental work done. This delay gives your vital force more time to be strengthened by homeopathy. In the case of emergency dental work, have it done and call your homeopath afterwards. In a dental emergency, homeopathic remedies will often relieve the pain until you have a chance to visit your dentist.

Recreational drugs: Avoid all recreational drugs including marijuana, cocaine, LSD, barbituates, and amphetamines. Alcohol in moderation is not a problem.

Other homeopathic remedies: Except in a first-aid situation, do not use them without discussing them with your homeopath first.

Herbs: Check with your homeopath before using herbs for specific medicinal purposes. Herb teas for beverage use, when varied from day to day, are fine, as are culinary herbs. If you've been given *Natrum muriaticum,* you will usually be advised to avoid menthol and peppermint in all forms, including tea. For other patients, peppermint is generally not a problem. There may be other specific substances that your homeopath will ask you to avoid when taking a particular remedy.

Vitamins: Let your homeopath know which vitamins you are taking. Using a particular vitamin to eliminate a particular symptom may make it difficult for your homeopath to evaluate your symptoms. Multivitamins and minerals are generally compatible with homeopathic treatment.

Permanent waves: These may interfere with remedies because of the harsh and aromatic chemicals used.

Other therapies: Acupuncture and therapeutic ultrasound have been known to disturb homeopathic treatment in some cases, although both may also have significant therapeutic value. Please discuss these therapies with your practitioner.

Factors Which Do Not Interfere with Homeopathic Treatment

Medications: We have not seen aspirin, acetaminophen, ibuprofen and other nonsteroidal anti-inflammatory medications interfere with homeopathic treatment.

Heating pads and water bed heaters.

Medical tests: Blood tests, x-rays, mammograms, Pap smears.

Dental examination and cleaning.

Cleaning products: Ammonia and bleach.

Personal care products: Most toothpastes, aftershaves, and deodorants that are not strongly aromatic are fine. Soaps, perfumes, and colognes that do not contain the substances listed above are rarely any problem.

Therapies: Massage (using nonaromatic oils), chiropractic adjustments and other forms of bodywork are generally compatible with homeopathy. If your complaints are primarily in your muscles and joints, it is best to discuss the frequency of these treatments with your homeopath.

The Patient's Freedom During Homeopathic Treatment

It is natural when starting anything new to have a period of adjustment. Avoiding some things like coffee or your electric blanket, which are important to you, or postponing dental work or your next permanent wave appointment may seem like a big imposition when you are just trying homeopathy for the first time. If your homeopath asks you to avoid certain things, you may feel that he places too many restrictions on your life and makes you feel rebellious.

Most patients who choose homeopathy find that it becomes relatively easy to avoid these substances and that allowing their remedies to work over time is well worth the effort. They find that the better health and increased freedom in their lives resulting from homeopathy is more important than the freedom to drink coffee or use camphor.

Your homeopath does not want to restrict you without good reason. When the remedy you need is clear and it has definitely worked for you, you may be able to use some of the things which you have avoided if they do not interfere with your individual treatment. The most crucial time for avoiding antidoting factors is before your homeopath has evaluated the effectiveness of the prescribed remedy. If the remedy does not get a sufficient chance to act because of an antidoting factor, your symptoms may not improve. If your homeopath interprets this lack of improvement as an incorrect prescription and changes remedies, the correct medicine may be abandoned too soon.

If you feel too restricted by your homeopathic treatment, discuss this with your practitioner. Perhaps you are avoiding some substances unnecessarily. If a potential antidoting substance is important to you, discuss using it in a controlled way, noting the results. If your symptoms return or become worse, you can stop using it and your homeopath can give you another dose of remedy if you need it.

Give your homeopathic treatment a chance to work. In a chronic case, it may take several months before the correct remedy has been found and has produced definite improvement. You can play an important role in your treatment success by carefully following your homeopath's instructions and being patient with the process.

Many patients who are treated homeopathically are so satisfied that they continue to use homeopathy for the rest of their lives.

WHAT DO I NEED TO KNOW ABOUT HOMEOPATHIC TREATMENT?

THERE IS A DEFINITE COURSE of treatment that homeopaths follow with their patients. This includes the number and frequency of follow-up visits, when to change or repeat a homeopathic remedy, how to deal with interfering factors, and what to do in case of an emergency. All of these depend on the symptoms, prognosis, and circumstances of the individual patient.

How Soon Will I Notice a Response to My Remedy?

You may notice an immediate response from your homeopathic remedy, as in the following case:

Jody

Jody, age 6, came in because of left-sided ear pain. She was so lethargic that she remained curled up in her mother's lap during the entire half hour interview. She was fair-skinned with long blonde curly hair and blue eyes. Since she developed the ear pain, she was very weepy and wanted to be with her mom all of the time. It was a struggle to get her to drink anything. She was given *Pulsatilla* (wind flower) in the office. Within five minutes she was running around happily and said that her ear pain was gone. She looked like a normal, healthy child again.

In other cases, it may take several weeks or a couple of months after taking your remedy before you notice a change in your symptoms. The length of your treatment depends on many factors, including the severity of your illness, the clarity of your symptoms, your past medical and family health history, the type of treatments which you have had in the past, and the overall strength of your body's defenses. Acute diseases, such as colds, flus, pneumonia, and bladder infections respond very quickly to homeopathy and will usually be cured in a few hours or one to two days. In chronic illnesses, such as arthritis, allergies, asthma, uterine fibroids, and colitis, it may take longer to respond to the remedy. After you take your remedy, you may experience a brief worsening of your symptoms. This is called an *aggravation*. Most aggravations last from a few hours up to several days. If an aggravation occurs, it is probably a normal part of treatment and usually means that the correct remedy has been given.

Symptoms that you have had in the past may recur during the course of homeopathic treatment. This is called the *return of old symptoms*. Usually they will last for a few days, then recede. It is as though the body were remembering, then repairing, an old illness. Often these symptoms will not return again.

Homeopathic treatment is analogous to both peeling an onion and digging up weeds by the root. If you are trying to clear a blackberry patch to plant a garden, you need to eradicate the plants at the roots. Cutting back the vines is only a temporary solution. Homeopathy heals by finding and curing the roots of disease. As symptoms from the past appear, your homeopath will recognize a layer of illness as it comes to the surface to be healed, or a predisposition that needs to be eliminated. She will prescribe a remedy that matches the symptoms of the layer. This process continues until all the layers, even back to your childhood and your hereditary predispositions, have been removed. During this process, you may continue to need the same homeopathic medicine, or you may need different remedies, depending on your state of health.

Sunita

Sunita, age 25, heard about homeopathy from a close friend whose hay fever had been cured. She suffered from chronic allergies and hoped that she could be helped, too. Because of her particular emotional state and allergy symptoms, she was given *Nux vomica*. This remedy made the allergy symptoms 80 percent better. Three months later, Sunita had a flareup of her eczema, which had been suppressed with hydrocortisone cream since childhood. She had terrible itching and was awake all night scratching herself raw. She felt very hot in bed at night. These symptoms are characteristic of homeopathic *Sulphur*. After receiving *Sulphur,* Sunita had an aggravation of the eczema for two months. She had a strong belief in homeopathy and her homeopath assured her that the flareup of the eczema was necessary for her healing to be completed. Afterwards her eczema was 90 percent better and the improvement has continued.

How Do I Know If The Remedy is Working?

Four to eight weeks after you take your remedy, your homeopath will evaluate the results of the prescription at the first follow-up visit. There are specific criteria which he uses to evaluate your response to a homeopathic remedy, including how much energy you have, whether your chief complaint is better, and whether you are better mentally and emotionally. By comparing your current symptoms with how you were before the remedy, he decides what to do next. He looks for what has changed and what has stayed the same in your case. It may be obvious to you that you have improved, but sometimes our memories are long for pleasure and short for suffering. You might be surprised when he reminds you of all of the symptoms you reported before you took the remedy.

Kristy

Kristy sought treatment for her chronic headaches and anger. During the initial interview, she stated that she had suffered from headaches every single day of her life. On her return visit five weeks later, we asked how she was doing. She replied that she wasn't sure. She had not noticed a change in her anger. Yet she had not experienced one single headache, for the first time in over forty years. Kristy had quickly forgotten how debilitating her chronic headaches had been. She had been given *Nux vomica,* a remedy for both headaches and anger. As her homeopath suspected, by the time of her next visit two months later, her anger had diminished considerably.

What If My Progress Seems Too Slow?

If you have a chronic illness, there may be times when you feel impatient and want more immediate results from homeopathy. It is useful to remember how long it took to develop the illness and to understand that the healing of chronic illness may take time. It is unrealistic to expect that you will be completely better in a few days when you have suffered from an illness for years. Homeopathic healing is cumulative. A patient who continues with treatment for more than a year generally finds that her overall level of health improves considerably. Her complaints become more minor. Instead of having asthma, she may only experience a mild bout of hay fever. Rather than the suicidal depression she experienced before homeopathy, she may have only an occasional day of "the blues."

Barbara

Barbara began homeopathic treatment twelve years ago. At that time, she complained of terrible headaches, premenstrual syndrome which nearly incapacitated her, and asthma. She was married to a man who constantly put her down. She wanted desperately to leave the marriage, but didn't feel strong enough to do so. She responded very well to a succession of homeopathic remedies. Over the first few years after starting treatment, her premenstrual symptoms, asthma, and headaches improved. After four years, she left her husband and felt much happier. She found a more lucrative job, which she liked much better. A couple of years later she started a relationship with a man who treated her tenderly and was very supportive. She has had no problems with asthma for seven years. For the past few years, her homeopath has seen her only two or three times a year for periodic episodes of neck stiffness and pain and mild premenstrual symptoms. She has been given remedies for these symptoms and felt better within days. She is happy with her life, feels good, and has few colds or minor illnesses.

How Often Will I Need to Take a Remedy?

Your homeopath will determine when you need to take a remedy based on your progress. She will decide whether or not to repeat or to change your remedy. *It is important that you return for your scheduled appointments at specified intervals, even if you are doing well,* so that your practitioner can carefully evaluate your progress and see if a new remedy or potency is needed. Follow-up appointments are usually scheduled every one to six months, depending on how you are doing. If, for some reason, it is impossible for you to return for a follow-up visit, at least write to your homeopath so she knows what is happening with you and how the remedy has affected you. Many homeopaths are willing to do phone interviews if an in person visit is not possible. Do not be surprised if your homeopath decides to wait weeks or months before prescribing another remedy. More harm is likely to be done by giving a remedy too soon than by waiting too long, or by changing the remedy before the first remedy has completed its action.

Prescription Drugs and Homeopathy

If you are taking prescription drugs when you first see a homeopath, he may prescribe the homeopathic remedy in low potency daily doses. This often involves a delicate balance of gradually decreasing the dosage of your prescription medication as your symptoms are improving, with the guidance of the prescribing physician. If you have taken thyroid medications for years or are on heart medication or insulin, you will probably need to remain on these medications, as your physician prescribes them, for the rest of your life, with or without homeopathic treatment. Another alternative is to wait to begin your remedy until nonessential medications are stopped so that there will be no confusion between the results of starting the remedy and stopping the prescription drug. This requires coordination between the patient, the homeopath, and the prescribing physician.

Some homeopaths will not treat patients on allopathic drugs, because they think that prescription medications make the prognosis less favorable. The majority of homeopaths, however, will treat you despite the drugs you are taking. Certain drugs may not be compatible with homeopathic treatment, including antibiotics, steroids and chemotherapeutic drugs when used on an ongoing basis. Any medication that suppresses the symptoms the body is trying to express is likely to interfere with homeopathic treatment. The two treatments may work at cross purposes. One example of this is the use of birth control pills specifically to treat irregular periods and menstrual discomfort. By preventing ovulation, the real symptoms of menstruation may be masked, making the task of finding the correct homeopathic remedy difficult or impossible. The same is true if you are taking drugs to suppress a discharge or a skin eruptions. This may be the outlet that your body needs for healing and these drugs may thwart that process.

Will I Have to Take a Homeopathic Remedy Forever?

Yes and no. As long as you are well, or in the process of changing for the better, you may not need a remedy for months or even years. Homeopathy makes you more resistant to disease, but life is stressful and you may not stay well forever, even if your homeopathic treatment has been effective. If you develop new symptoms or your old symptoms return, it is important to check in with your homeopath to see if you need to be treated again. Many patients who are treated homeopathically are so satisfied that they continue to use homeopathy for the rest of their lives.

When Should I Contact My Homeopath?

If you develop an acute illness that needs treatment. Call your homeopath *before* seeking other forms of treatment for acute illnesses. If you have a medical emergency such as a car accident, severe bleeding, heart attack, stroke, or poisoning, get emergency medical treatment immediately, then call your homeopath as soon as possible. If you have rapidly progressing acute symptoms such as an earache, pain when urinating, or an unusually bad cough, call your homeopath immediately. If you cannot reach your homeopath, seek conventional medical care for severe acute illnesses.

If you think that you have been exposed to one of the substances that interfere with homeopathic treatment. Your homeopath may wait one to two weeks before re-evaluating your case and deciding whether to repeat your remedy. This waiting period is sometimes necessary to evaluate whether your previous symptoms return and to give you a chance to recover without the need for repeating the remedy.

If you think nothing has happened from the remedy and you want to use another form of treatment to alleviate your symptoms. You may not have waited long enough to feel the full effect of the remedy you have been given, or another remedy may be needed. In either case, using another treatment before the action of the remedy has been evaluated may confuse your case. Your practitioner may be able to recommend something that will alleviate your discomfort yet will not interfere with your homeopathic treatment.

If you experience a severe aggravation after you take a remedy. This is unusual, but it can happen and your practitioner should know about it immediately.

If you experience significant symptoms that you have never had before These may come from the remedy you have taken or from another cause, but they need to be promptly evaluated by your homeopath.

If old symptoms return severely for more than two weeks. A return of old symptoms is usually mild and short lasting, but occasionally the situation needs evaluation and treatment.

If you want to use prescription medications that you have not already discussed with your homeopath. This includes antibiotics, steroids, anti-inflammatories, hormones and other strong prescription drugs that may disturb your treatment.

If you need to have dental work or surgery. If it is an emergency and you can not reach your homeopath, have the work done. If the dental care can wait, your homeopath may have a preference as to *when* the dental work is least likely to interfere with your homeopathic treatment.

If you need extensive diagnostic procedures. Invasive diagnostic interventions such as exploratory surgery or other procedures may affect your treatment. You should use these diagnostic techniques when necessary, but let your homeopath know.

If you do not know when to come in for your next follow-up appointment or you are unsure whether to continue homeopathic treatment. Your homeopath can guide you to the most appropriate next step in your healing process. If homeopathy has not worked well for you, which is occasionally the case, your homeopath may refer you to another homeopath or to a different type of practitioner.

If you are traveling and need medical care. Your homeopath may be able to treat you by telephone, or to recommend a homeopath nearby. In emergencies, remedies can be sent by overnight mail or taken on your trip in a traveling kit. This is far better than to risk interfering with your treatment.

"I sank deeper into depression. It was at this time that I saw an article by a homeopathic doctor and decided that I would try, one more time, to get my life on an even keel... That was the best decision I have ever made."

REAL PATIENTS, REAL CURES

THE FOLLOWING ARE TRUE CASES from our clinical practice. All of the patients whose stories are told gave their permission and were eager to share their positive experiences with homeopathy. The names have been changed, as have all the other patients' names in the book, to protect privacy. The stories in quotations are told by the patients themselves. The others are narrative summaries of cases from our practice.

Cliff: Allergies

"It wasn't until I got better that I saw how sick I was. My typical day for most of my 36 years consisted of slowly waking from a not so restful sleep, feeling haunted by past events for most of the day, crashing, dog-tired, by four in the afternoon, and then going home to be alone. From time to time, I sneezed. At the time I thought my life was just like everyone else's, except I had allergies.

"I battled allergies since I was 14. A series of skin tests indicated I was allergic to tomatoes, dusts, trees, grass, and molds, all of which seemed unavoidable. I began taking injections of a dark syrupy substance that relieved the congestion and sneezing. After taking the injections for a few years, I concluded that I was cured.

"Unfortunately, a few years later my allergies not only returned, but were worse. I had not been cured as I had thought. Whatever it was inside of me that caused the allergies was still there. Was it genetic? I had never had a good relationship with my father and this gave me even more reason to resent him. After millions of years of genetic evolution, this was the best my body could manage?

"My medical doctors suggested surgical desensitization by scraping the nerve endings out of my nose. It seemed so barbaric. I had trouble believing that the nerve endings in my nose were the fundamental problem and I didn't want to lose a part of me that I couldn't get back.

"After considerable study on my part, I found that if I ate only rice and frozen vegetables and took seventy-five assorted pills each day I was fine. With my health under control, I turned my attention to working out my anger towards my father. At 33, I went to a few Adult Children of Alcoholics meetings and began to explore my past.

"My decision to seek additional help at this time was purely economic. I was spending a fortune on pills each month and wanted someone to help me determine which ones I didn't really need. I found my homeopathic doctor. I told him I just wanted to cut the inventory of vitamins, extracts, and unknown compounds I was taking. Ours was to be a short term relationship. I explained in extensive detail that poor nutrition, resentments about past events, and bad luck had conspired against me and resulted in allergies. I was sure that better nutrition was the answer.

"He listened to me a lot during that first appointment. Then, without saying much about my medicine cabinet full of pills, he gave me a little envelope filled with a small amount of white granules. He said it was a preparation of salt. I took it in the evening before bed.

"I woke the next morning from the most restful sleep I had had in years. To my disbelief, both of my nostrils were open and clear! I felt fifteen years younger, could breathe easily, and had high energy throughout the day. I was delighted to find that afternoon fatigue was not a typical part of the adult human experience. I also found that I could eat anything. And I did, with great relish. I no longer felt bloated or poisoned by foods that I ate.

"My body worked better and I felt that something deep inside had changed. It felt like a big tuning fork in my abdomen had been given a big whap. Every part of my body worked better. I no longer felt the need for the pills I was taking. It seemed like magic.

"Over the next few months I noticed that my attitude toward myself gradually improved. I was no longer as self critical and afraid of being hurt emotionally. I became more vulnerable. Then a few months after first taking the remedy I began to feel such deep emotions that I thought I was going crazy. The remedy seemed to nudge to life feelings that had been suppressed very deeply.

"I took the salt remedy, *Natrum muriaticum*, for about a year. I was very pleased with what was happening. My only complaint was that my case was apparently so simple and that something as basic as salt was the cure I had needed all along.

"I then felt some changes in my disposition. I began to sneeze again for the first time in months. I felt like a couch potato. I did not care to do anything or go anywhere. I found myself working obsessively and began to snap at people at work. I recalled an earlier period in my life that was very similar.

"My homeopath prescribed another remedy, *Nux vomica.* I no longer felt driven to work. My sneezing stopped once again. By the time I recognized that the intense anger I was feeling was part of the healing process started by the remedy, it was over.

"Over the five years I have been under homeopathic care, my life has improved steadily and dramatically. I am no longer held captive by the old negative feelings that guided my life. Allergies are no longer a problem. I can eat any food; I have more energy. Homeopathy helped me release my fears about intimate relationships, which enabled me to get married and have a child. My wife and daughter have also enjoyed the benefits of homeopathy."

Donna: Chronic Fatigue Syndrome

Donna was a bright 29 year old office manager who sought out homeopathy because she was tired. Really tired. She had been that way for close to five years. Donna loved to sleep. When she woke up in the morning, she was still exhausted and felt like she could sleep another two hours. She felt exhausted after work. Even when she wasn't working, she was still extremely fatigued at the end of the day. When Donna was tired, she felt like a cloud came over her. Her body felt like it just faded away and, before she knew it, she was asleep. She was too tired for sex. She was normally a very kind and gentle person, but when she was tired, she became defensive and grumpy.

Before the fatigue began, Donna was quite industrious and enjoyed cooking and gardening. She enjoyed her challenging job, but worked too hard. Donna didn't want to change jobs because she "wasn't a risk taker" and she had a fear of new situations.

Donna complained of severe, debilitating headaches. She had bowel movements only every three days. She was very chilly, especially her feet. She loved to wrap up in a blanket and be out in the sun. Her overall health had been good until the fatigue set in.

Donna was given *Silica* (sand). This is a homeopathic medicine for people who lack "grit." They just don't have the energy to respond to the demands placed upon them. They have desires and strong opinions, but it is just too much effort to act on them. They become very fatigued when they work too hard. Their nature is to be gentle, refined, and timid. They are chilly and often constipated like Donna.

After one month Donna reported that she was no longer exhausted, just normally tired at the end of the week, and she needed less sleep. She felt good when she woke up in the morning. Her mind was clearer. She had no headaches, and she was happy to report that her sexual energy was back to normal. Her body also felt warmer. Donna noticed that she stood up for herself more. Her newfound energy enabled her to enjoy her weekends again. She began sailing lessons, which she really enjoyed.

By six weeks after the homeopathic remedy, Donna's energy was back to normal and she no longer felt irritable. Even though she was under stress, she was coping quite well. Her improvement has lasted for more than two years.

Sally: Depression

"I decided to visit a homeopathic doctor after several years of battling depression. I was able to maintain an outward appearance of competency and appeared to deal with life, but inside I was fighting depression and deep feelings of inadequacy. Over the years I had been in counseling, had read all of the self help books I could find, and had reconnected with my spiritual beliefs. For the first time I truly felt that my life did make sense and that there was a reason to live. But the sadness and lack of self-confidence remained. Every avenue of self help that I tried would help for a short period of time, but the effect did not last. I felt at that time like I was on an endless pendulum. Each time it swung, I sank deeper into depression. It was at this time that I saw an article by a homeopathic doctor and decided that I would try, one more time, to get my life on an even keel.

"That was the best decision I have ever made. After several years of counseling and homeopathy, I have finally reached a point in my life where I feel good about myself. The effect of homeopathy was to stop the pendulum. Finally I have a feeling of quiet peace and joy about life, myself, and the people around me. I do not consider homeopathy the answer to the questions of life. What it has done is to reduce the endless feelings of fear which resulted in depression. It reduced my emotional swings to the normal variations in mood that everyone must experience. What is even more important, I now have enough peace to search and can take joy in that search for the answer to 'Why am I here?'"

Sonya: Menopause

Sonya, a 44 year old artist, had received homeopathic treatment periodically for years. During that time she was treated successfully for depression, headaches, and digestive problems. She consulted a homeopath because of anxiety that seemed to come on with menopause.

Sonya told her homeopath, "My brain has been used up. I feel pressure in my head. My mind does not want to function. I have burning hot flashes from the slightest excitement. They spread from my head and face to my whole body. My whole body sweats. My mind is constantly thinking about business. I wake frequently at night. I am always figuring things out during my sleep. I organize things in my mind for work. I'm always taking care of business.

"My fingers and arms get numb easily on waking. It is worse from sleeping on my left side. I have an aching sensation in my forearms and wrist, especially on the right side. It is almost a burning, but kind of feels icy cold and tingles. My lower eyelids, back and legs are twitching lately.

"I have a hurried feeling. It's overwhelming. There's not enough time. I have to tell myself to slow down. I can't think. It's an effort. Nothing connects. I lose my train of thought. I forget words. I get so speedy that I forget half of what I'm thinking about.

"I'm bloated and I have gas. My bowels are sluggish. I have an inner gnawing feeling. If I get hungry, watch out and don't get near me! I have a tightness in my larynx. It feels tense."

Sonya had had no menstrual period for the previous five months. She was generally much warmer since the hot flashes began. She couldn't find a comfortable sleep position because her mind was "chewing" all the time. She desired sweets and spicy food. She was thirsty for cool drinks. The sun and light were bothering her again lately and she noticed recently that she was more afraid of heights. Sonya was very anxious to feel better.

Sonya was treated with *Iodum* (Iodine). *Iodum* is a remedy for people whose metabolism is extremely high. They are hurried and restless. It is as though their engines were revved up to maximum speed. They feel they must be busy all the time and are anxious when they are quiet. They become very warm and can have flushes of heat all over the body, with red cheeks, and profuse perspiration. They often have voracious appetites, as Sonya did, as well as a tight feeling in the larynx and a gnawing sensation in the stomach.

Sonya called her homeopath several weeks after she took the remedy to say how well the remedy had worked. The rushed feeling in her mind and restlessness were gone within twenty-four hours. Within two weeks, she was "back on track." The hot flashes disappeared completely. The numbness in the fingers and arms was gone, as well as the aching of the wrist. These symptoms were still better two years later.

Lucy: PMS, Endometriosis, and Infertility

Lucy, a 29 year old realtor, sought out homeopathy because of years of endometriosis, an abnormal growth of uterine tissue outside the uterus. She had undergone laparascopic surgery a year and a half earlier to remove endometrial tissue in the area of the rectum and tailbone. She had been infertile for the previous three years and very much wanted a child. Lucy had a miscarriage shortly before coming to see us. She drank heavily during the pregnancy, but had been in recovery and completely free of alcohol since that time.

"My PMS is ridiculous. I get really aggravated. I feel angry inside. I try not to take it out on others, but I think they're idiots! I get angry even at the way my husband breathes. I snap at him. If he asks me to make a decision, I'm short. I say, 'Don't ask me.' or 'Give me my space.' I'm like this for about ten days every month. I feel better a few hours after my period arrives."

Lucy had plenty of premenstrual symptoms: "I have massive water retention. My eyelids get puffy and my abdomen bloats. My breasts get really sore. My uterus feels heavy, like a rock. I have uterine pain during sex before my period. My sex desire goes down with the PMS. I get low back pain, too. It is as if all the blood is drawn out of my back. I get a sharp pain inside my rectum before my period and during a bowel movement if I bear down.

"I was bulimic for about five years. I didn't have any periods for four of those years. Then, for three years, I flowed heavily for three or four days. I had to put in a tampon every hour or two. My periods are okay now, except my uterus hurts when I put in a tampon. My bulimia lasted from age 19 to 25. I only ate a small amount of cottage cheese every day, then I vomited at night. From age 21 to 26, I drank all day. I started drinking when I was 17. I drank hard liquor for the first four years, then cheap white wine. I would drink half a gallon in two days.

"My knees are often sore. I can only stand in one spot without moving for about five minutes. I have to crack my knees often. It's hard to sit in movies or a car. It's as if my knees don't fit where they're supposed to. I've been this way since I was 12. My knees are worse the day before it rains. They ache. I can't crawl around on my knees."

Lucy complained of little sores inside her nose. They felt like cuts. A couple of her teeth turned black as a child. Her wrists had always been weak.

"I'm chilly. My extremities are cold, but I don't like the heat. It makes me cranky. I can't stand saunas or hot baths. I broke my ankle about five years ago. When it snows, it really hurts." Lucy slept on her left side. She was diagnosed with an iron deficiency starting at age 12 and often took iron supplements.

Lucy was usually easy going and relaxed. It was hard to put herself in new situations, but once she did, she was fine. She had a great fear of spiders. She would sweat, shake, and become paralyzed if she saw a spider on TV. She couldn't even talk about them. She had fears of her husband leaving her.

"I was 12 when my parents separated. It was horrible for me. My world blew apart. There were four of us. That's when I started doing drugs. I quit high school in my senior year and got my G.E.D. My father is still alcoholic. My mother is from an alcoholic family. All three of my siblings are in recovery. I've been married five years. I get very jealous. I can be too sympathetic with people. I want to fix it for everyone. Then I berate myself when I can't."

Lucy received *Calcarea phosphorica* (calcium phosphate), an important remedy for PMS, bone and joint weakness and pain, and dental problems, all related to an inability to assimilate calcium. It is also a remedy for menstrual or hormonal problems beginning at puberty, for anemia, jealousy, and is a common remedy for knee pain as well as for incomplete healing of fractures.

At her next visit, five weeks later, she reported that she had no emotional symptoms before her period. The premenstrual breast tenderness was mild. Sex was pain free. The shooting rectal pain was gone. She hadn't had a premenstrual time this easy in years. "Is this too good to be true?" she asked. Her husband couldn't believe it. He asked Lucy in disbelief, "Is it here already?" She did not gain her usual five to seven pounds before her period. She had absolutely no premenstrual irritability. Her knees were a little better. Her energy was increased. She was less jealous. She felt remarkably better.

When Lucy consulted her homeopath four months later, her main complaint was nausea of pregnancy! She was very excited about being pregnant, after three years of unsuccessful efforts, but felt horrible all the time. "It's as if I have the flu, but I don't throw up." She had nausea from the moment she woke up in the morning. It was worse around 2 to 3 p.m. "I feel like I'm gonna die." The nausea was worse from laughing, from the smell of car exhaust, smoke and coffee. Her sexual energy was "zip" since she became pregnant. Her breasts were tender.

In addition, some of Lucy's old symptoms were back. She felt the sharp pain in the rectum again. She was angry with her husband like before the remedy. The low back pain had returned over the previous two days. She experienced a little twinge of jealousy one day for the first time since the remedy. Lucy was given another dose of *Calcarea phosphorica* because her symptoms still matched this remedy picture. This was four and a half months after the original dose.

Lucy called her homeopath a week later to say she was feeling much less nauseous. Her energy level was a little better. Her sex drive was coming back. She was feeling less irritable. Now, over three years later, she has a healthy daughter who also receives homeopathic treatment and Lucy continues to be very healthy.

Helen: Eczema

"Over the past four years, I had seen eight medical doctors in my attempt to cure my eczema. The medical doctors prescribed drugs and ointments that were as debilitating, physically and emotionally, as the disease itself. They told me, 'You'll have to learn to live with it' and 'Maybe you should see a psychologist.' I did as I was told to do by the medical doctors, but it only suppressed the symptoms and did nothing to cure the disease. My skin was so bad I even had thoughts of suicide. My quality of life became the issue. I am so glad I looked for help once more and tried homeopathy.

"It's a miracle. I can wear clothes. I can sleep. I can be comfortable all day without drugs or medicated ointments. These statements bring tears of joy to my eyes. I had suffered from skin eruptions and constant, uncontrollable itching. I had open, weeping skin wounds. My scratches became so infected that I still have scars all over my body."

Gina: Arthritis

Gina, 72 years old, had suffered from arthritis all her life. When she was a child her mother had always told her she wasn't strong, which had angered her. Gina's knees hurt from age 12 until her 20's, when she became pregnant. She had always had weak ankles and had turned them frequently in the past. Now she was stooped over with osteoporosis.

At the time of her first homeopathic visit, she complained of heaviness and tension in her low back. It felt "all bound up." It was worse on first getting up and better from loosening up. By noon everyday Gina felt tired and she would nap after lunch. She felt that she just didn't have enough energy. Gina's knees hurt to walk. Putting weight on them gave her a sharp pain, especially her left knee. This caused her to lose her balance. She complained of upper back pain when she was tired and experienced a continuous pain between her shoulder blades. This pain was better if she lay down for fifteen minutes with her knees up. At age 52, she had a successful laminectomy to relieve sciatic pain. She complained of having always had "lousy hair and nails."

Gina was a raw foods vegan and felt this was the only correct way to eat. She had been constipated all her life until she began eating raw foods exclusively. She had a healthy appetite, but never gained weight. She had been manic depressive in her 30's and took lithium carbonate for eight years. She had an early menopause at age 39. She tried estrogen for a few years.

Gina had a problem with insomnia. She often woke between two and four in the morning. The insomnia was worse if she was worried or upset. Her sleep was not very sound. It was hard for Gina to relax. She felt a sense of anxiety in her stomach, like "butterflies." She hated deadlines, but she was extremely punctual. She didn't like it when other people were late. Gina was quite neat and did not appreciate her roommate's sloppiness. She was very sensitive to the cold and felt chilly even in warm weather.

Her homeopath gave Gina *Kali carbonicum* (potassium carbonate), a prominent homeopathic arthritis medicine. It is helpful for people who suffer from pain in the low back and shoulder blades and who wake between two and four a.m. Pain in the knees is also common in people needing this medicine, as well as a sensitivity to cold weather and a feeling of anxiety in the stomach or solar plexus. They are often quite proper, with fixed ideas about how things ought to be. Gina's stringent dietary regimen, punctuality and fastidiousness are typical of the rigid way in which someone needing *Kali carbonicum* might think.

At her first follow-up appointment, one month after the remedy, Gina said she felt much better. She was sleeping well and felt much warmer. Her joint symptoms were much better. She was not having pain in the lower back, knees, ankles, or the upper back. Her energy was greatly improved.

By the time of the second visit, five weeks later, Gina reported that she felt better with every passing day. Her joints still did not hurt. She had gained a few pounds and was 118 now. Her ankles felt stronger. She commented, "I'm better now than I have been for a long time." Her hair and nails had grown much stronger. She felt that she was able to express her feelings much more freely, and she was more accepting of herself. Gina's arthritic symptoms have continued to improve.

Carlos: Obsessive Jealousy

"I have suffered chronic back pain and persistent stomach problems for the past sixteen years. I have also had kidney stones several times in my life. Some stones required surgery; others were removed with a great deal of discomfort. As a result, I learned to deal with pain firsthand.

"I also learned to deal with adversity early in life. I was born in a humble rural community in Puerto Rico. My mother died when I was 10 years old. I was the oldest of seven children. We were separated after my mother's death. Our home was destroyed and we were sent to live with different relatives. I experienced hunger and hardship.

"Last summer, for no apparent reason, I became extremely despondent and depressed. I found no comfort in my loving family. Their love had brought me so much joy before. Now I felt as if they didn't need me and didn't care if I lived or died. In reality, nothing could have been further from the truth, but this is how I felt. I became insanely jealous of my wife without cause. I wished for my death with each sunrise and sunset. I can find no words to adequately express what I was feeling at that time.

"In this state of mind, I met my homeopathic doctor. Unfamiliar with alternative medicine, I was a little apprehensive, but so desperate that I was willing to try almost anything.

Within a few months after beginning homeopathy, I started experiencing subtle changes in my personality and my thinking. I developed a new, positive outlook on life and felt rejuvenated. I was able to release much of my insecurity, intolerance and impatience. In the past, I excused my bad temper with the simple alibi that I have a Latin temper. I don't need this excuse anymore. I enjoy a sense of serenity which I never before experienced. The formerly indispensable bottle of antacids in my nightstand has been replaced with classical music tapes. I have never felt so good."

Charles: Flu

Charles, age 61, sounded desperate when he called. His homeopath asked him to come in immediately. He looked awful. He was very weak and it was difficult for him to climb the flight of stairs to the office. He complained of a recurrent fever with chills over the previous ten days. His fever, about 102 degrees Fahrenheit, would begin at five or six p.m. and last until about four a.m. He was extremely confused, which was quite unusual for him. He had no appetite and had lost twenty pounds in two weeks. All he wanted to do was lie down. He had no energy or interest for anything, which worried him a great deal. His wife, who brought him in for his appointment, was also quite concerned.

Charles received *China* (cinchona bark), to take every four hours until he felt better. *China* is an important homeopathic medicine for great weakness and for fevers that periodically go up and down at consistent times. Charles called the next day to say he was feeling better. He had more energy, the diarrhea stopped, his mind was clearer, and the fever did not last as long the night he started the *China*. He called the following day to say all of his flu symptoms were markedly better. He was much relieved and his appetite was back.

We hope these stories of homeopathic cures will motivate you to seek homeopathic treatment for yourself and your family, and to stay with treatment until you receive the benefits you desire. These inspiring case histories show the kinds of improvement you might expect during your own treatment. Homeopathy can help you change your life and health in dramatic ways. Since homeopathy treats the whole person, positive changes may occur on any level, physical, mental or emotional. The cases in this chapter and throughout the book indicate only a few of the conditions for which homeopathy is useful. Consult with your homeopath to find out what kind of results you might expect from homeopathy in your case.

A well-trained homeopath has spent hundreds or thousands of hours learning homeopathy, often in addition to years of prior medical training. Mastery of homeopathy is not something that can be acquired in a few weekend seminars or even in practicing for a couple of years.

How to Find
the Right Homeopath

The Legal Status of Homeopathy

Certification through examination is offered by the American Institute of Homeopathy for medical doctors and osteopaths (DHt) and the Homeopathic Academy of Naturopathic Physicians for naturopathic physicians (DHANP). There is no specific licensing for homeopaths in the United States except in Arizona, Connecticut and Nevada. The North American Society of Homeopaths (NASH) and the Council for Homeopathic Certification (CHC) are establishing standards for unlicensed professional homeopaths in the United States and Canada with the ultimate goal of licensure.

Laws regarding the practice of homeopathy vary from state to state. Homeopathy can be practiced in most states, depending on the licensure of the practitioner. Naturopathic physicians are licensed to practice homeopathy in Arizona, Alaska, Connecticut, New Hampshire, Hawaii, Montana, Oregon, Washington, Nevada, Florida, and the District of Columbia. They also practice in many other states where licensure efforts are under way. It is important that practitioners and the public inform their legislators and state medical associations that they want continued access to homeopathic medicine.

Choosing Your Homeopath

Most homeopathic practitioners have a degree, are licensed in a health care profession, and have taken postgraduate training in homeopathy. Some lay or professional homeopaths do not have formal medical training, but may be highly skilled in homeopathy. A well-trained homeopath has spent hundreds or thousands of hours learning homeopathy, often in addition to years of prior medical training. Mastery of homeopathy is not something that can be acquired in a few weekend seminars or even in practicing for a couple of years.

One important factor in choosing a homeopathic practitioner is the level of experience. Find out what percentage of her practice is devoted to homeopathy and if homeopathy is her primary method of treatment. Most serious homeopaths will devote at least 50 to 75 percent of their practices to homeopathy, even if they also use other therapies. Homeopaths improve with experience. If you have a complicated condition, you may wish to find a practitioner who has specialized in homeopathy for at least five years. Even if you have to travel to see a well-trained, experienced homeopath, the results will likely be well worth it. We and many other homeopaths are willing to do long distance phone consultations since there are many areas without trained homeopaths.

Directories of homeopaths in the United States are published by the International Foundation for Homeopathy and The National Center for Homeopathy. A directory of naturopathic physicians who are board certified in homeopathy is available through the Homeopathic Academy of Naturopathic Physicians.

Are There Different Kinds of Homeopaths?

Practitioners who follow the principles of Hahnemann are said to be *classical* homeopaths. Classical homeopaths conduct the type of extensive interview we have mentioned and base their prescription on all of the symptoms that the patient relates during the interview. They prescribe only one remedy at a time, based on the law of similars. We strongly recommend that you find a classical homeopath for the most effective and long lasting results. If you have any doubt as to whether a particular homeopath follows a classical approach, ask that question specifically. If you are still uncertain, select a homeopath listed in one of the directories mentioned above.

Practitioners who use electrodiagnosis, auricular therapy, pendulums, radionics or kinesiology to determine the correct remedy may use homeopathic medicines, but they are not practicing homeopathy as it was developed by Hahnemann. They usually prescribe many remedies in combination and do not base their prescriptions on careful selection of the one remedy that best matches the patient's symptoms.

How Can I Tell If I Am Seeing The Right Homeopath?

The criteria that you use for determining if your homeopath is right for you are personal, but the following general guidelines may be useful:

Does he listen to you and to your concerns?

Does she seem interested in your progress and well-being?

Are you improving from the treatment?
Is your chief complaint better? Have you improved mentally and emotionally? Is your energy and vitality better? Are other symptoms improving? Is your improvement generally following the laws of cure?

Have you been treated for a long time without success?
If there is no improvement after six months to one year of treatment, perhaps it is time to find another prescriber or ask for a consult or a referral to another homeopath. If you decide to change to another practitioner, discuss your decision with your present homeopath.

Does he behave unethically or abusively to you in any way?
Abuse or unethical behavior is never appropriate in the homeopathic process.

Does she inform you about your treatment and prognosis?
Honest communication between homeopathic practitioner and patient is essential.

Do you usually have to return for visits more often than monthly?
It is unusual that your homeopath would need to see you more than monthly, except for very serious chronic illness, acute illnesses, or emergencies.

Does he keep complete and confidential records?
This is important not only to accurately document your clinical progress, but also for insurance and legal purposes. If you decide later to switch to another homeopath, a transfer of your complete homeopathic treatment history is important.

Homeopathic treatment can open a door to a healthier life. You have the choice whether or not to walk through the door and make the changes in your life that will prevent the same patterns of illness from emerging again.

MAKING THE MOST OF
YOUR HOMEOPATHIC TREATMENT

It's Never Too Late

The best time to start homeopathic treatment is now. It does not matter what your health problems are, how old you are, how many doctors you have seen, what treatments you have already tried, and what has and has not worked for you. Your homeopath will work to understand where you are now and what can be done to help you. Homeopathy cannot benefit you if you are still on the fence, wondering if you should try it. We can only encourage you to give it a try and make the most of what homeopathy can do for you.

The Role of Homeopathy in Your Life

Life, health, career, and relationships are all subject to change. How you adapt to the changes impacts your well-being and provides an opportunity for personal growth. Homeopathy *cannot* prevent every illness or trauma that you may experience in life; but homeopathy *can* help you maintain the energy, physical well-being, clarity of mind, creativity, and equanimity that you need to learn the most from and cope with the ups and downs of life.

Homeopathy is a wonderful tool for regaining health and maintaining balance in your life. As with any tool, how you use it is up to you. Homeopathy can treat severe chronic illness, or simply help you to heal a sprained ankle or get over a cold or the flu. At whatever level you choose to use it, homeopathy can help. For those of you who are interested in treating yourselves and your families, we hope you understand the importance of seeking care from a professional homeopath for chronic illnesses, and only treating minor conditions on your own.

The best way to maximize the benefits of homeopathy is to use it as part of an integrated lifestyle including a loving and supportive network of family and friends, challenging and meaningful work, a healthy diet and exercise program, and a spiritual life which brings you peace and joy. Homeopathic treatment can open a door to a healthier life. You must choose to walk through the door and make the changes in your life that are necessary to prevent the same patterns of illness from emerging again.

Your Responsibility as a Patient

Your understanding of the homeopathic process and your willingness to follow the guidelines given to you by your practititioner can make a big difference in the success of your treatment. You have a vital role to play in the process. You have the power to use homeopathy in many ways to enhance your well-being. It is not just in your homeopath's hands, but in yours, too. Take an active role in your treatment. Observe yourself and your symptoms. Ask questions. Be aware of your response to the treatment and tell your homeopath about it. It is your responsibility to call or see your homeopath regularly and whenever questions or problems arise. It is up to you to be aware of those influences that may interfere with your homeopathic treatment and to avoid them. Your participation is vital to your success with homeopathy.

The most important contribution you can make towards success in treatment is to stay with the process over months and years. As your overall health improves, you will need fewer office visits, but regular follow-up will help you remain healthy. An astute homeopath can observe slight changes in your health and adjust your treatment before any significant illness occurs. Prevention is an essential part of the homeopathic process, just as important as treating your acute and chronic illnesses.

Our Goal and Your Goal

Our goal in writing this book is to help as many of you as possible to experience the benefits of homeopathy and to live healthy, happy lives. If your goal in reading it is to understand homeopathy better so that you can get well and stay well, please use the information we have given you to truly make the most of your homeopathic experience. We hope all of the guidelines and suggestions we have offered throughout the book do help you to better understand and make use of this fascinating art and science.

Whether homeopathy is an entirely new philosophy of medicine for you or you are a seasoned homeopathic patient, there is always more to learn. Reading this book is a good beginning. Other books, articles, classes and courses are available to expand your knowledge. For those of you who just can't wait to learn more about it, we offer the following resources for further exploration.

Appendix:
Learning More

Recommended Books

General Interest

Bellavite, Paolo and Signorini, Andrea. *Homeopathy: A Frontier in Medical Science*. Berkeley: North Atlantic, 1995.

Castro, Miranda. Stress: *Homeopathic Solutions for Physical and Emotional Stresses*. London: Macmillan, 1996.

Johnston, Linda. *Everyday Miracles*. Van Nuys: Christine Kent Agency, 1991.

Jonas, Wayne B. and Jacobs Jennifer. *Healing with Homeopathy: The Complete Guide*. New York: Warner Books, 1996.

Reichenberg-Ullman, Judyth and Robert Ullman. *Ritalin-Free Kids: Homeopathic Medicine for ADD and Other Behavioral and Learning Problems*. Rocklin: Prima Publishing, 1996.

Ullman, Dana. *The Consumer's Guide to Homeopathy*. New York: Tarcher/Putnam, 1995.

Ullman, Dana. *Discovering Homeopathy: Your Introduction to the Art and Science of Homeopathic Medicine*. Berkeley: North Atlantic, rev. 1991.

Self-Treatment

Castro, Miranda. *The Complete Homeopathy Handbook*. New York: St. Martin's, 1990.

Castro, Miranda. *Homeopathy for Pregnancy, Birth, and the First Year*. New York: St. Martin's, 1992, 1993.

Cummings, Stephen and Ullman, Dana. *Everybody's Guide to Homeopathic Medicine*. New York: Tarcher/Putnam, rev. 1997.

Kruzel, Tom. *The Homeopathy Emergency Guide*. Berkeley: North Atlantic, Homeopathic Educational Services, 1992.

Panos, Maesimund and Heimlich, Jane. *Homeopathic Medicine at Home*. New York: Tarcher/Putnam, 1980.

Ullman, Dana. *Homeopathic Medicines for Our Infants and Children*. New York: Tarcher/Putnam, 1992.

Ullman, Robert and Reichenberg-Ullman, Judyth. *Homeopathic Self-Care, The Quick and Easy Guide for the Whole Family*. Rocklin: Prima, 1997.

For the Homeopath or Serious Student

Agarwal, M.L. *Materia Medica of the Human Mind*, Sixth edition. Delhi: Pankaj Publications, 1993.

Barthel, H. and Klunker, W. *Synthetic Repertory*. New Delhi: B. Jain, 1990.

Boericke, Wm., M.D. *Materia Medica with Repertory*. Santa Rosa: Boericke and Tafel, 1927.

Coulter, Catherine R. *Portraits of Homeopathic Medicines*. Three volumes. Berkeley: North Atlantic, 1986.

Coulter, Harris. *Divided Legacy: A History of the Schism in Medical Thought*. Vol 3. Berkeley: North Atlantic, 1981.

Hahnemann, Samuel. *Organon of Medicine*. Sixth edition, 1842. Reprint. Los Angeles: J.P. Tarcher, 1982.

Herscu, Paul. *The Homeopathic Treatment of Children: Pediatric Constitutional Types*. Berkeley: North Atlantic, Homeopathic Educational Services, 1991.

Julian, O.A. *Materia Medica of New Homeopathic Remedies*. Oxford: Beaconsfield, 1979.

Kent, James T., *Lectures on Homeopathic Philosophy*. Berkeley: North Atlantic, 1979.

Kent, James T., *Lectures on Homeopathic Materia Medica*. Reprint. New Delhi: B. Jain, 1982.

Kent, James T., *Repertory of the Homeopathic Materia Medica*. Reprint. New Delhi: B. Jain, 1991.

Morrison, Roger. *Desktop Guide to Keynotes and Confirmatory Symptoms*. Albany: Hahnemann Clinic, 1993.

Moskowitz, Richard. *Homeopathic Medicines for Pregnancy and Childbirth*. Berkeley: North Atlantic, 1992.

Phatak, S.R. *Materia Medica of Homeopathic Medicines*. New Delhi: Indian Books and Periodicals Syndicate, 1977.

Sankaran, Rajan. *The Spirit of Homeopathy*. Bombay: Homeopathic Medical Publishers, 1991.

Sankaran, Rajan. *The Substance of Homeopathy*. Bombay: Homeopathic Medical Publishers, 1994.

Schroyens, Frederik, ed. *Synthethis: Repertorium Homeopathicum Syntheticum*. London: Homeopathic Book Publishers, 1993.

Tyler, M.L, *Homeopathic Drug Pictures*. Devon: Homeopathic Research and Educational Trust, 1952.

Van Zandvoort, Roger, ed. *The Complete Repertory: mind*. Leidshendam: Institute for Research in Homeopathic Information and Symptomatology, 1994.

Vithoulkas, George. *The Science of Homeopathy*. New York: Grove, 1980.

RESOURCES

Homeopathic Book Distributors

Homeopathic Educational Services
2124 Kittredge St.,
Berkeley, CA 94704
(510) 649-0294

Homeopathic Informational
 Resources, LTD.
9099 Oneida River Park Drive
Clay, NY 13041
(800) 289-4447

The Minimum Price
250 H St., PO Box 2187
Blaine, WA 98231
(800) 663-8272

Pacific Homeopathic Books
 and Supplies
7028 120th St., Suite # 205
Surry B. C. V3W 3M8 Canada
(604) 572-8879
Fax (604) 591-2349
(800) 572-7765 (orders only)

Homeopathic Organizations

American Institute of
 Homeopathy
1585 Glencoe
Denver, CO 80220
(303) 321-4105
Journal: *Journal of the American Institute of Homeopathy*

American Homeopathic Pharmacists Association
PO Box 174
Norwood, PA 19074

Foundation for Homeopathic
 Education and Research
2124 Kittredge St.
Berkeley, CA 94704
(510) 649-8930

Homeopathic Academy
 of Naturopathic Physicians
PO Box 69565
Portland, OR 97201
(503) 795-0579
Journal: *Simillimum*
Conference transcripts for sale.
Directory of Practitioners

Homeopathic Pharmacopoeia
 of the United States
PO Box 40360
4974 Quebec St. N.W.
Washington, D.C. 20016

International Foundation for
 Homeopathy
PO Box 7
Edmonds, WA 98020
(206) 776-4147
Fax (206) 776-1499
Journal: *Resonance*
Professional Courses
Directory of Graduates
Annual Case Conference
Conference Books and Tapes

The National Center for
Homeopathy
801 N. Fairfax, #306
Alexandria, VA 22314
(703) 548-7790
Fax (703) 548-7792
Journal: *Homeopathy Today*
Directory of Practitioners and
Study Groups available.

North American Society of
Homeopaths
10700 Old County Road 15
Plymouth, MN 55441
Journal: *The American Homeopath*

International Homeopathic Organizations

British Homeopathic Association
27 A Devonshire Street
London, W1N 1RJ England
Journal: *Homoeopathy*

The European and International
Councils
for Classical Homeopathy
ECCH and ICCH Secretariat
School House, Market Place
Kenninghall, Norfolk
NR16 2AH, England
Tel/Fax: 011 44 953 88 163

The Faculty of Homeopathy
Royal London Homeopathic Hospital
Great Ormond Street
London, W1 1DF, England
Journal: *The British Homoeopathic Journal*

Hahnemann Society
Avenue Lodge,
Bounds Green Road
London N22 4EU, England

Journal: *Homoeopathy Today*

The Homeopathic Education
Society
Natakkar Gadkari Road, Irla,
Vile Parle (West)
Bombay 400 056, India
Journal: *Indian Journal of Homeopathic Medicine*

Homoeopathic Links
De Ree 11
9753 BX Haren
The Netherlands
31 (0)50-5347101
Fax 31 (0)50-5347101
Journal: *Homeopathic Links*

Liga Medicorum
Homeopathica Internationalis
P.O. Box 66, 2060 AB
Bloemendaal, Netherlands
Journal: *Journal of the LMHI*

Pan-American Homeopathic
Medical Congress
Edificio 166, Entrada D.
Unidad Kennedy, México 9, D.F.

Society of Homeopaths
2 Artizan Road
Northampton, NN1 4HU
United Kingdom.
Journal: *The Homoeopath*

Homeopathic Pharmacies

Ainsworth's Homeopathic
Pharmacy
39 New Cavendish Street
London W1M 7LH, England
011 44883340332

Boericke and Tafel, Inc.
2381 Circadian Way
Santa Rosa, CA 95407
(800) 876-9505 (West Coast)

Boiron USA
98-C W. Cochran St.
Simi Valley, CA 93065
(800) BLU-TUBE
or 6 Campus Blvd. Bldg. A
Newtown Square , PA 19073
(800) 876-0066

Dolisos America, Inc.
3014 Rigel Ave.
Las Vegas, NV 89102
(800) 365-4767

Ehrhart and Karl
2419 N Ashland Ave.
Chicago, IL 60614-2020
(800) 607-7447

Hahnemann Pharmacy
828 San Pablo Ave.
Albany, CA 94706
(510) 527-3003

Homeoden
Kasteellaan 76-9000
Ghent, Belgium
011 91 25 87 33

Homeopathy Overnight
4111 Simon Rd.
Youngstown, OH 44512
(800) ARNICA 30, ext. 140

Luyties Pharmacal Co.
4200 Laclede St.
St. Louis, MO 63108
(800) 325-8080

Propulsora Homeopatía
de México
Calle Mirto 116 y 118
México, D.F. México 06400

Standard Homeopathic Co.
210 W. 131st St., Box 61067
Los Angeles, CA 90061
(800) 624-9659

Washington Homeopathic
Products, Inc.
4914 Del Ray Ave.
Bethesda, MD 20814
(301) 656-1695
(800) 336-1695 (orders only)

Homeopathic Software Organizations

CARA
Christopher Jayne
Chiron
P.O. Box 424
Port Townsend, WA 98368
(360) 385-1917

HomeoNet
Institute for Global
Communications
18 De Boom St.
San Francisco, CA 94107
(415) 923-0900
or Kent Homeopathic Associates

MacRepertory and ReferenceWorks
Kent Homeopathic Associates
PO Box 39
Fairfax, CA 94978
(415) 457-0678

RADAR
Homeovia
P.O. Box 56603
8601 Warden Avenue
Markham, Ontario L3R OM6
(800) 668-7543

Homeopathic Training Programs

Academy for Classical Homeopathy
7549 Louise Ave.
Van Nuys, CA 91406
(818) 776-0078

Bastyr University
14500 Juanita Drive, N.E.
Kirkland, WA 98034
(425) 823-1300

Four Winds Seminars
187 Hillside Drive
Fairfax, CA 94930
(415) 457-8452

Hahnemann College
of Homeopathy
828 San Pablo Ave.
Albany, CA 94706
(510) 524-3117

International Foundation for
Homeopathy
P.O. Box 7
Edmonds, WA 98020
(425) 776-4147
(425)776-1499 (Fax)

National Center for Homeopathy
801 N. Fairfax, #306
Alexandria, VA 22314
(703) 548-7790

National College of
Naturopathic Medicine
049 S.W. Porter
Portland, OR 97201
(503) 499-4343

New England School of
Homeopathy
356 Middle Street
Amherst, MA 01002
(203) 763-1255

Pacific Academy of Homeopathic
Medicine
1678 Shattuck Ave. #42
Berkeley, CA 94709
(510) 549-3475

The School of Homeopathy
(Devon, England)
The New York Center
for Homeopathy
41 E. 57th St., #1606
N.Y., NY 10022
(212) 570-2576

GLOSSARY

acute illness – a condition which is self-limiting and short-lived, generally only lasting a few days to a couple of months.

aggravation – a temporary worsening of already existing symptoms after taking a homeopathic remedy.

allopathic medicine – treatment of disease through using drugs which produce opposite effects, such as conventional medicine.

antidote – a substance or influence which interferes with homeopathic treatment.

artificial disease – an illness which is given to a person intentionally, in the form of a homeopathic medicine, in order to overpower the already existing disease.

case taking – the process of the in-depth homeopathic interview.

centesimal – a type of preparation of homeopathic medicines which is based on serial dilutions of 1 to 99, designated by the letter "C".

chief complaint – the main problem which causes a patient to visit a health care practitioner.

classical homeopathy – a method of homeopathic prescribing in which only one remedy, based on the totality of the patient's symptoms is given at a time, followed by a period of waiting to evaluate the action of the remedy.

combination remedy – a mixture containing more than one homeopathic medicine.

common symptoms – those signs and symptoms which are common to any person carrying a particular diagnosis.

constitutional treatment – homeopathic treatment based on the whole person, involving an extensive interview and careful follow-up.

decimal – a type of preparation of homeopathic of homeopathic medicines which is based on serial dilutions of 1 to 9, designated by the letter "X".

defense mechanism – that aspect of the vital force whose purpose is to maintain health and defend the body against disease.

empiricism – a method of scientific inquiry which is based on observation and experience.

general symptoms – those symptoms pertaining to the body as a whole.

Hering's law of cure – the principle that cure occurs from the top to the bottom, from the inside out, from the most important organs to the least, and in the reverse order in which the symptoms presented.

high potency remedies – remedies of a 200C potency or higher.

homeopathic medicine – a medicine which acts according to the principles of homeopathy.

homeopathy – the use of the same substance which causes a particular set of symptoms to relieve those same symptoms.

HPUS – the standard homeopathic pharmacopeia of the United States.

law of similars – the concept that like cures like.

low potency remedies – remedies of a 30C potency or lower.

materia medica – a book which includes individual homeopathic remedies and their indications.

mechanism – a type of scientific thought which views the individual as a machine whose individual parts can be understood and repaired.

miasm – an inherited or acquired layer of predisposition.

minimum dose – the least quantity of a medicine which produces a change in the patient.

modality – those factors that make a particular symptom better or worse.

mother tincture – the initial, standardized alcohol preparation from which homeopathic dilutions are subsequently made.

nosodes – homeopathic medicines made from the products of disease.

particulars – those symptoms pertaining to an individual part of the body.

polychrest – a widely used homeopathic medicine which treats many symptoms.

potency – the specific strength of a homeopathic medicine determined by the number of serial dilutions and succussions.

potentization – the preparation of a homeopathic remedy through the process of serial dilution and succussion.

prover – a person who takes place in a systematic experiment of taking a particular medicine for the purpose of eliciting symptoms.

proving – an experiment in which a substance or medicine is taken repeatedly and the effects carefully documented.

relapse – the return of symptoms when a homeopathic medicine is no longer acting.

remedy – a homeopathic medicine prescribed according to the law of similars.

repertory – a book which lists symptoms and the medicines known to have produced such symptoms in healthy provers or in patients.

return of old symptoms – the re-experiencing of symptoms from the past after taking a homeopathic medicine.

rubric – a symptom listed in a repertory followed by a list of the medicines which may produce this symptom in a healthy person and may relieve the symptom in a patient.

Schuessler cell salts – a collection of twelve low potency homeopathic remedies which are taken individually or in combination.

simillimum – that one medicine which is nearest to the totality of the symptoms of the patient and which will produce the greates relief.

single remedy – one single homeopathic remedy given at a time.

succussion – the systematic and repeated shaking of a homeopathic medicine after each serial dilution.

suppression – the elimination of a particular symptom without the vital force being strengthened, and sometimes being weakened.

totality of symptoms – a comprehensive picture of the whole person: physical, mental, and emotional.

vital force – the invisible energy present in all living things which creates harmony, balance, and health.

vitalism – the philosophy of science which imbues each living organism with an all-pervading energy force.

INDEX

ABOUT THE AUTHORS

Robert Ullman, N.D. received his B.S. in Biology from Ursinus College and did graduate study in psychology at Bucknell University. He graduated from The National College of Naturopathic Medicine with a Doctorate in Naturopathic Medicine in 1981. He was formerly chair of homeopathic medicine at Bastyr University. He is currently Vice President of the International Foundation for Homeopathy (IFH).

Judyth Reichenberg-Ullman, N.D., M.S.W. graduated with a B.A. in Spanish Literature from George Washington University and a Master's in Psychiatric Social Work from the University of Washington. She received her Doctorate in Naturopathic Medicine from Bastyr University in 1983. She is President of the IFH.

Both Judyth and Robert are licensed naturopathic physicians and board certified members of the Homeopathic Academy of Naturopathic Physicians. They are cofounders of The Northwest Center for Homeopathic Medicine in Edmonds, Washington where they are in private practice, specializing in homeopathic family medicine. They are available to treat patients by telephone consultation if there is no homeopath in your area. Their office telephone number is (425) 774-5599. Visit their website at http://www.healthy.net/jrru for their speaking and teaching schedule, articles and homeopathic audio tapes on Healthworld Online .

They are instructors in the IFH Professional Course and teach and lecture widely. Authors of *Ritalin-Free Kids: Homeopathic Medicine for ADD and Other Behavioral and Learning Problems,* and *Homeopathic Self-Care,* they are also columnists for *Resonance,* the publication of the IFH and *The Townsend Letter for Doctors and Patients.* You can contact them for speaking engagements at Picnic Point Press, 131 3rd Avenue, N. Suite B, Edmonds, WA 98020. Tel: (206) 233-1155. Fax: (425) 670-0319.

Robert and Judyth reside with their two lovable golden retrievers in Edmonds, Washington, which overlooks beautiful Puget Sound and the Olympic Mountains.

ORDER FORM

Please send me

___copies of *The Patient's Guide to Homeopathic Medicine.* $10.95

___copies of *Ritalin Free Kids.* $15.00

___copies of *Homeopathic Self-Care.* $18.00

___*Homeopathic Self-Care Medicine Kit (50 Homeopathic Medicines) $80*

20% discount on 5 or more copies, plus shipping and handling.

Name: _____

Address: _____

City: _____State: _____ Zip: _____

Telephone: (   ) _____

VISA/MC number: _____

Exp. date: _____ Signature: _____

Shipping and Handling

$3.50 for the first book; $1.00 for each additional book. $5.00 per kit. Washington residents, please add 8.6% sales tax. Allow 30 days for delivery.

Telephone or Fax Orders

Call (206) 233-1155. Leave a message with your name, address, telephone number, Visa/Mastercard number and expiration date, and quantity ordered, or fax this order form to (425) 670-0319.

Mail Orders

Please fill out credit card information or make checks payable to:
Picnic Point Press
131 Third Ave., N., Suite B
Edmonds, WA 98020